Happy Naked

A straight-forward, five-senses guide to loving the skin you're in and feeling that energy in every area of your life.

By Denise Mago

To Deborah, Valery, and Hector
You are my sunrise and my sunset.

And, to all those who
hunger for the naked truth.

Table of Contents

The Naked Truth 1

Why this book works 5

Being Fit Doesn't Mean Being Perfect 9

THE DEE-5 System of Holistic Health...................... 14

Section 1: Getting Started

How to Make This Book Work for You 17

The Naked Truth about Time 24

Feeling Your Way to Change 28

Section 2: Getting A Move On

Restorative Sleep 36

In Real Life What Will You Do? 47

Supportive Nutrition 58

The Naked Truth about Nutrition.............................. 60

Easy Meals That Can Create Sustainable Habits...... 78

Complete Excercise 94

Sharp Mental Health 119

Tranquil Soul_ 131

Section 3: Tying It All Together

Syncronicity 144

Tracking Your Happy Naked Life 164

Acknowledgements 168

About the Author 171

The Naked Truth

Is there a voice in your head telling you to look away from your reflection because you're just not perfect enough?

When people say how nice you look, do you tell them all the reasons why you don't deserve that compliment?

Do you turn the lights off during times of intimacy or shy away from nakedness all together?

There have been many times in my life when I had that little negative voice inside, too. During, and especially after, my three pregnancies was when I fully understood my relationship with my body. The one thing that benefited me most was that I was very active, so my fitness level was really good for being pregnant.

As a health and fitness professional, I used to put a lot of pressure on myself to lead by example like having that hard-body look expected of a fitness expert. All that focus on external perfection caused a huge rollercoaster in my inner and outer health when I experienced an unknown illness in December 2016 that affected my body, my emotions and my mind.

Between 2014 and 2017 I went from being in the best shape of my life to being in the worst shape of my life. I was experiencing an illness that no specialist could figured out and the pain was taking my happiness away. I was prescribed medications and with that came side effects such as skin issues, gut issues, weight gain and circumstantial unhappiness.

My body felt like it belonged to someone else. Physical pain mounded right on top of emotional pain. I was most definitely not Happy Naked. Most people close to me didn't really notice because I appeared fit on the outside. But when I looked in the mirror, all I could see, and especially feel, were the imperfections in my naked body.

What got me through was my belief that everyone deserves to feel at home in their body--even me. I had seen my fitness clients transform their lives when they took care of their whole selves. This was the birth of my DEE-5 System of holistic healing.

At the core of the DEE-5 System is a belief that every facet of a person is connected. You cannot heal the soul without also nurturing the body. You cannot build strength without also resting deeply. You cannot be truly Happy Naked without deeply caring for every part of your body and your inner self.

Being Happy Naked means being comfortable with your own vulnerability. It means feeling truly confident in your own body. When you are Happy Naked, you don't need to have sex with the lights off. What's sexy opens up to include all that is intimate, sensual, kinky, romantic, long and slow, or quick and wild.

As I've been developing and practicing my DEE-5 System, I am getting more and more deeply in love with my body. The older I get and the more my body and hormones change, the more vital it is that I am happy with my naked body, my naked personality and my naked spirit.

When the intimacy in YOUR life gets to the next level (and it will!) your confidence will be there. That comfort in your own skin will also encourage you to bring your life, career and relationships to a level you truly deserve.

You will achieve a greater good that benefits yourself, your family, your work and ultimately the planet earth that needs so much love and care.

This book will propel you toward finally being HAPPY in your own NAKED body. Are you ready?

Let's dive in!

Why This Book Works

Small books fit in purses. Reminiscent of little books of faith, small books packed with life-changing information are today's version of the common book of prayer—this one is the common book of the senses. Unlike electronic versions, small books made of paper can be touched, smelled, seen, even heard and tasted. And they can be doodled on and written in.

The purpose of *Happy Naked* is to inspire life-altering change: the kind that leaves the shadow of your former self in the dust. The kind where your dream-image of yourself and your life appear before you, in the mirror, each morning.

This small book is with you for the long haul. Change takes time but, make no mistake, the smallest of changes made today means you will never be the same as yesterday, and the smallest changes made over time are the most impactful.

This book is separated into three sections.

Getting Started

Five senses and change: this part is where you are given the idea of how self-love and self-improvement will be different this time because of an indulgence of your senses.

Getting a Move On

A motivational 'go for it, do your thing' to make your life shine: the part where each key area of life is defined, and where help, tips, suggestions, and direction (plus some questions) appear in abundance.

Tying it All Together

A way to see where you fit: a practical way to be inspired through stories of those who were dealt frustrating circumstances, met those challenges by making changes, and came out stronger for it. And a suggestion to track your year ahead.

All the stories in this book are based on those of real people. I have changed their names and identifying details to maintain their confidentiality. I am so grateful to know them and to have their permission to share their inspiring stories with you.

Gain Access to Exclusive *Happy Naked* Resources

I know from helping hundreds of people, having multiple types of tools and resources is invaluable to a transformation journey. I have created an entire webpage full of journal pages, videos, exercise tips and more – just for you, my dear *Happy Naked* warriors. I will keep adding to the page over time.

To gain access to all this goodness go to
http://deehealthnfitness.com/resources/
password: 8xxx8

***def:* DEE-ism**

Dee Mago's wellness philosophies advocating

Determination, Empowerment, and
Encouragement

involving five elements and the five senses.

Latino Zen + Naked Truth

Being Fit Doesn't Mean Being Perfect

Do we need to be told—through media or in person—how to live life? The healthy, confident answer is 'no way!' An expanded option could be, 'Only if we ask how to live our life.'

The sad thing is that we *do* let others tell us how to eat, drink, dress, spend our leisure time and generally behave. Media bombards us with uninvited *you ought to do this, buy that, feel this* all the time. On the negative side, we permit media to erode our boundaries and our sensibilities.

On the positive side, thank goodness, we have mentors: women of wisdom, men of benevolent kindness, elders who reset our core values, proactive humanitarians, and goddess warriors who led us to the greatness that exists within each of us.

Mentors don't tell us how to live our lives; they show us how to get the most out of the life we have been blessed with.

Take my situation, growing up in Venezuela in a family of strong women. Right from birth, I created memories with my great-grandma, my grandma, my mom and my sister.

My Abuelita (little grandma) raised my sister and I while my mom studied. She continued to care for us when my mom worked to provide for us. My dad was an infrequent presence. From an early age, through the journeys of these amazing women, I was raised to be an empowered female throughout my childhood.

At eleven years old, I got to step into my own strength and be my Abuelita's greatest company and support, in the night, when she would wake and cry over the death of one of my uncles. Seeing her suffering from grief, I decided to help find her another purpose to distract her from the pain: a job at my school as an English teacher. I convinced her to go to an interview that I had personally arranged with the principal. She got the job. That life-changing event for her created a ripple effect throughout our community.

I am who I am because of the strong women I was raised by.

Love and humour create life. During our last family reunion, my Abuelita looked at all of us and said "I am so proud to have a family of good-looking people. There is not an ugly person here." I burst out laughing at her comment. We all need to love and to laugh, and that includes loving ourselves and laughing at ourselves. Quirkiness is underrated, as is self-love and deep-laughter.

Mostly, though, my heart soared, because my Abuelita's definition of 'good looking' means that we are happy, healthy, strong, confident, and loving.

This book is about identifying the 'good looking' in *you*. We make choices about whole, healthy living at every age. And that form of 'good looking' is the most attractive form of human-ness.

Women are born leaders. We raise families, form groups of friends, support co-workers, care for the young and the old. Here's to resilience, intelligence, and forward thinking.

The idea that each of us is not 'media perfect' is absolutely perfect in my opinion. Unique circumstances create unique individuals. The collective ideas of those individuals change the world. That is how culture emerges. Those cultures, filled with communication in the form of dance, meals, rest, respect of space and personal boundaries, build individual success.

We each inhabit our own world. Notice I did not say little. That's because our worlds are not little. We each inhabit a *massive* world that is filled with cells. Some even say that a whole universe exists within each cell. Our energies reach deep within, to a place we each call 'me.' Those energies reach out to mentor, hold space for, and honor all those who are also in their own adjoining worlds, like dancing with ourselves and the whole world at all times.

I love that common bond, an infinite way of looking at celebrating life. I love that we are each the choreographer, the dancer, the music, the stagehand, the usher, the ticket taker, and the audience all at the same time.

On that note, this book is a little longer than one of those old-fashioned dance cards our grandmothers or other grandmothers have spoken of, yet much shorter than an encyclopedia of 'you are broken, here's how to fix your life.' Happy Naked is a little book of my philosophy, my way of sharing and caring with you, the love I have learned to give to myself, thanks to my gracias *Abuelita*, and in turn, have already shared with hundreds of women in a collective journey.

I propose that a healthy life is created by including gems and treasures from five components I call the DEE-5 System of Holistic Health, which you will experience through your senses. In the end, life is about more than looking good naked, it's feeling truly *Happy Naked*, inside and out.

THE DEE-5 System of Holistic Health

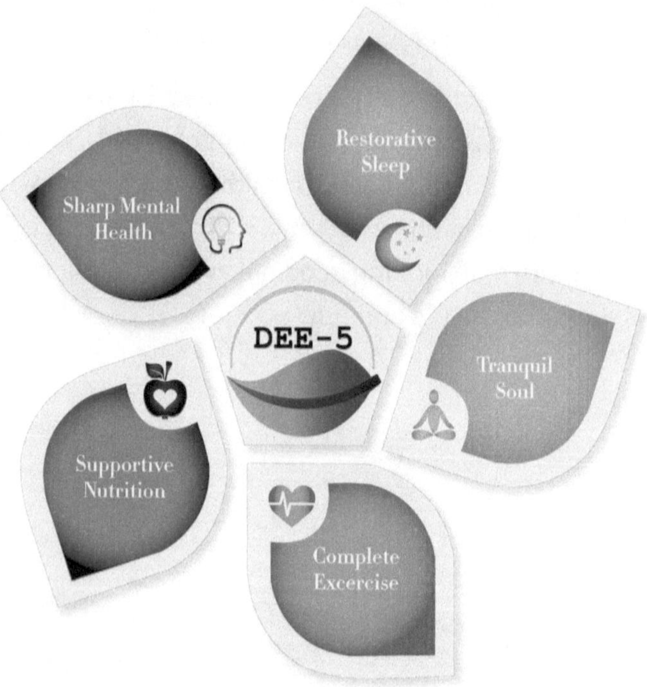

In a nutshell, here are the five-to-thrive components of a healthy life:

RESTORATIVE SLEEP: – seven to eight hours a night.

SUPPORTIVE NUTRITION – no diet, consideration of organic and non-GMO.

COMPLETE EXERCISE – fun, challenging, consistent.

SHARP MENTAL HEALTH –less stress, balanced, realistic scheduling, knowledge.

TRANQUIL SOUL – spirituality, gratitude, forgiveness, deeper thoughts.

AND CONNECT TO YOUR 5 SENSES IN ALL AREAS OF GROWTH AND CHANGE

1) Feel / Touch

2) Look / See / Vision

3) Taste

4) Smell

5) Sound

SECTION 1
GETTING STARTED

How to Make This Book Work for You

Build from where you are right now. Begin with the basics. The most transformative actions to implement in moving through your *Happy Naked* journey are outlined in this easy-to-follow program. You will be creating new habits, making healthier choices and feeling better in your own skin as you work through each section of the book.

Pro-tip: Work with yourself as a whole person, not just a physical body.

And keep challenging yourself. You need your body to be 100% healthy to perform in life at full potential.

Incorporate the Five-To-Thrive

Work with at least one component from each of the DEE-5. Understand that all the sections work together, in combination. Using only one or two sections compromises the full experience and reduces success rates.

Drill Down

Focus on a habit you know is not serving you, then select something from each section that will help you overcome that habit. Make sure to take that habit and write how it tastes, sounds, looks, feels and smells. Then take the opposite of the habit and apply the same senses. Feel that contrast. Aim for the enhanced senses.

Write For Success

Journal, even if it's one phrase or a doodle in the middle of the page. It could easily be your descriptions of the senses applied to words you choose. Write in the margins. Draw stick women. Whatever feels good. Journaling is cathartic: it satisfies the brain and supports mental health. It guides the soul, soothes the self, helps in recognizing habits, changes dreams to goals to the realization of those goals, tracks the journey, and is ultimately a celebration of ***YOU***.

Take a Holistic Approach

Living a healthy life is absolutely doable when we combine elements from each of the DEE-5 System instead of focusing on only one. Put simply, using tools and devices from each category keeps us balanced: we neither fall over, nor fall off.

You know when someone is in love and goes 'all in' as in 'experiences all the senses?' Well, full immersion in the DEE-5 System produces an even better love high than that feeling. That's because it's for, and with, your 'Self,' not someone else. Who better to love than yourself?

The challenge is how to blend these five categories and prioritize them in your life every day. In the DEE-5 System we do this by applying our senses: touch, sight, taste, smell and sound. When we do this, the results are amazing because we're immersing our whole self into the experience—we bring our whole self to the table of life.

It's true: positive messages reach every cell when we actively examine how each of the DEE-5 categories feels, looks, tastes, smells and sounds.

Healthy Life Visualization

Journal your answers to the following visualization questions:

What does a healthy life look like to you? Is it a single color, more than one, or, if framed, what is the scene?

Does it have a flavour? What does healthy life taste like?

Is there a scent to a healthy life?

What do you hear when a healthy life speaks?

How does it feel to your fingertips?

Examples to Kickstart Your Thinking

Here are some examples of how healthy life can be defined by using the five senses. Note: the descriptions are as unique as the person describing the life.

For one individual, the idea of a healthy life **appears** as a green meadow with multi-colored flowers peering above the grass. Lining one side is a row of blackberry bushes, the branches bending with a bounty of ripe fruit that is heavily **scented** like old, sweet wine. The

flavour of grandma's fruit crumble is on the tip of the tongue. Outside the frame, a bubbling stream (**sound**) hints at clear, pure, water. Arms outstretched, the air has substance and **texture**, as if it is an invisible but feel-able silk curtain.

For another, a healthy life **resembles** a room with a comfortable sofa, a full bookshelf, and an open window looking out onto the ocean. The **scent** of salt and sand filter through the window screens. The waves, crashing loudly at night, such **volume**. A fresh sheet of paper is lifted from a desk, smooth to the **touch**; the hand tingles as the page anticipates ink. It is impossible for the memory not to **taste** clams and mussels served with freshly baked bread, garlic, and melted butter.

Applying senses to describe one's whole life and playing with impressions, is a clear way to engage in a relationship with the self.

But what if our senses tell us a negative story? Sometimes things can taste sour and smell like rotting fish — that's okay too. Those are signs that 'stuff' is out of balance in our life. We have to see, taste, smell, hear, and touch them to move past them.

*****

At this point I hear some of you—maybe most of you—are full of questions. So let's get you some answers.

QUESTION: *Dee, you want me to get all poetic over five areas called DEE-5? Five areas with five senses, that's twenty-five things I don't have time for. I just want to lose weight.*

QUESTION: *It sounds interesting, but I thought this little book would 'tell' me what to do to fix things. I didn't grow up with all that support you had, and I don't have it now. How will this work for me?*

ANSWER: I hear you. You both sound frazzled and frantic, as if you are running from some kind of vengeful force. Please, stop. There is no one chasing you. That thing behind you that appears to be on your tail *is your tail*.

All I'm asking, at this point, is for you to get ready to use your imagination to describe what a 'healthy life' (and other concepts) looks, sounds, feels, tastes, and smells like—simple!

QUESTION: Dee, you're a sweetheart and totally motivating. You changed my friend Angie's life, but that is her. I'm not as perky as she is. She doesn't have children and I have three under ten. I don't know if I can…well, I don't have a great track record.

You are not Angela, and Angela is not you. Yet, we are all human and we all experience fear as a visceral presence. Angela learned that she could choose to deal with her fear by using her senses. You have the same senses as Angela.

We are our own monster under the bed. The enemy at the gate. The critic that tears apart our daily performance. We are. It's heartbreaking how cruel we are to ourselves.

We've all heard it before: We'd never say to another what we say to ourselves.

*****

The Naked Truth about Time

Ultimately, you know how much time you have in a day and a night. You know where it goes. If you're unclear on this, look back over the last twenty-four hours. If you truly cannot nail time wasters, then pick a day and make a diary on what you are truly doing with all that time.

At some point, if your social media time is balanced, your routine is relatively well organized, and you still have no time left over, then you might want to evaluate.

What can be delegated?

What can be dropped?

We live in a society where busy-ness is worn as a badge of honor

Sometimes we want an escape, but we feel guilty by having 'a break', so we find ways to numb out (social media, shopping, binge-watching TV, gaming). That numbing out time can add up, and because of the guilt associated with it, it's not enjoyable and calming. We are good at sneaking in time-outs because we think we shouldn't say we are doing 'nothing.' Consider the following suggestions to shift your thinking.

- Reevaluate

- Put you first

- Get rid of expectations; instead, set intentions

- Respond rather than react

- Breathe

- Simplify

- Delegate

Some of you might be breathing a little calmer now. You knew there were things within your sunrise to sunrise that you didn't really need to do, didn't want to do, didn't have to do, right?

- You knew your kids could walk to school.

- You knew you didn't have to go on Facebook thirty-seven times a day.

- You knew one old episode of Property Brothers would lead to a binge.

Now that you recognize that, you can shift some things. Most of us feel it will be difficult, if not impossible, to change our circumstances, but it doesn't have to be that way. Be gentle with yourself. Rome wasn't built in a day!

Leaning-In To Being Gentle With Yourself

1) You only need do a small amount, as little as you want. Small changes made over time are more impactful because they have staying power.

2) This 'work' is only done once. It is leading you to give your brain information about yourself.

3) Once the brain is 'awakened', any internal changes will become automatic. You have done the preparation by going through the sections and understanding the DEE-5 System. Once you 'get it,' you've got it for good.

4) If you want to add additional layers to your understanding and your experience, you can. You choose.

We often gather a bunch of things we want to be and do from reading and listening to others. This creates our 'personal list', our 'want list' or some might say 'bucket list.' Along the way, we add more dreams and desires, then we hit the wall. FEAR. Fear of change. Fear of commitment. Fear of starting now.

Starting what? Life? We're already living and breathing.

Change is scary. Even when it's a change to a smoother, more fun, more fulfilling life. Change creates fear of the unknown, and because we haven't changed anything yet, the fear is there. Hopefully it's accompanied by excitement or anticipation of something good. 'Fear of the Unknown' is the older cousin of 'Might Not Be Up For It.' I hear from these two all the time. These characters put pressure on us. They love it when we're too afraid to move past the point of 'want' and into the place of decision and action.

Feeling Your Way to Change

Rather than trying to defy fear, try aligning with it. By simply attaching senses to your fear, and then coming up with the opposite of fear and adding senses to that word, you'll be able to move through fearful thought patterns.

Below is an exercise in visualizing your fears. The reason for this exercise is that, ultimately, you have to look under your own bed. You will need to go to the gate with a flashlight. Get into the habit of using all your senses, so you can apply your senses to all your decisions and actions.

Visualization to Shine a Light on Your Fears

Take the word fear and describe what it smells, sounds, feels, tastes, and looks like to you in this moment.

Then, take a word that describes the opposite of your fear and apply the senses to that word.

The contrast is profoundly powerful. Can you feel the difference?

To access a guided meditation about visualizing your fears by Rick Titan (ricktitan.com) go to http://deehealthnfitness.com/resources/   -
password: 8xxx8

You'll also need to stop hurling insults at yourself. Those comments that you would never say to anyone else will become fewer as you immerse yourself in the five elements.

Real People. Real Visualizations.

Here are some examples of how others applied their senses to their brand of FEAR, and what they chose as the opposite of FEAR.

SANDRA on FEAR and her opposite: COURAGE.

"Fear tastes like overcooked Brussels sprouts; smells like them too. It sounds like my mother-in-law's 'I told you so' which echoes my own mother's rants, which brings in my father's tirades about politics (the tone more than the words). Fear looks like a slightly open door to a room at an aunt's house that my sister told me was haunted. It feels cold. Like I imagine a dead body might. That might be the body that died in the room my sister told me was haunted. There is no body, I don't even have an aunt—where did all that come from?"

Breathe in. Out. In. Out. It's alright…

"COURAGE! That's an opposite of FEAR. It's me, Sandra, tasting freedom by eating dark chocolate after having said 'no' to going to my mother-in-law's monthly supper. It sounds like Celine Dion—I don't care if others think she's overrated—The Power of Love at full volume in my car while it sits, with me in it, in the automated carwash. It looks like hiking boots and good waterproof socks at the base of a mountain. It feels like the inside of a sleeping bag—all warm.

Here. I. Come.

Watch. Out. For. Me.

I'm still a little bit scared, but bring on the chocolate. Saturday, when the family gets over their shock of having to toast their own bread, they'll survive, and I'll be hiking and facing fear."

Love, Sandra

BRIAN on FEAR and his opposite: ABUNDANCE

"FEAR is scarcity. It tastes like rice and beans. It appears as empty cupboards; smells like stale bread. It has the texture of rough blankets. It howls like coyotes a bit closer than they should be.

The opposite of fear, for me, is abundance. It looks like friends gathered at a restaurant. Tastes like a well-stocked fridge at home. Smells 'new clothes' clean—

no hand-me-downs. To touch abundance is to grip the handles of my bike and ride it along a mountain trail.

Listen! I hear laughter."

Thx, Bri!

JULIE on FEAR and her opposite: BLISS

"I shiver. He's coming for me. I smell his aftershave. Must comply. Or Hide. Fear looks like the underside of the mattress and bedframe. I am the non-monster hiding under the bed, avoiding the monster who rules the house. It sounds like constant orders: have you made your bed (is it all about the bed?), brushed your teeth, done your homework, practiced piano, said your prayers? It tastes like burgers. Wow, really? But it does. Fast food eaten in the car on the way to dance, swimming, tutoring. It tastes like rushing around on a diet of 'must dos.' It feels like leather upholstery—it feels like must keep up with so-and-so, they have a Land Rover."

"What the hell? Land Rover? Who had a Land Rover? The neighbors?"

"For me, the opposite of fear is bliss. I don't think I've ever used that word before. Bliss? I might have to look it up. Bliss—a state of utter contentment. Yes, I want to use that word. Bliss has the flavour of almonds as they might taste in the form of candy floss. It is silence. Clean, unadulterated peace and quiet. Pin drop. To touch bliss is to be submerged in a bubble bath so full that the water slops over the top of the tub. Effervescence from the tips of my toes to the top of my head and every place in between. It appears as an almost empty house, open plan, the ultimate minimalism—uncluttered, spacious, white, with candles in every room."

Love Julie

RICK on FEAR and his opposite: CALM

"Tastes bitter, like gall. Smells sweaty. Sounds like the rush of an approaching train. Fear looks like total darkness. To touch fear is to feel an indescribable object—I mean, it can't even be explained to one's self."

"The opposite of fear for me is calm. Sweet flavoured, the natural sugar of fruit. Its scent is a pine forest in summer. Calm announces itself as gentle waves lapping on the beach. To view calm is to see peaceful countryside from a hilltop. Stroking a resting animal, horse or dog, is what calm feels like to the fingertips."

Rick

SECTION 2
GETTING A MOVE ON

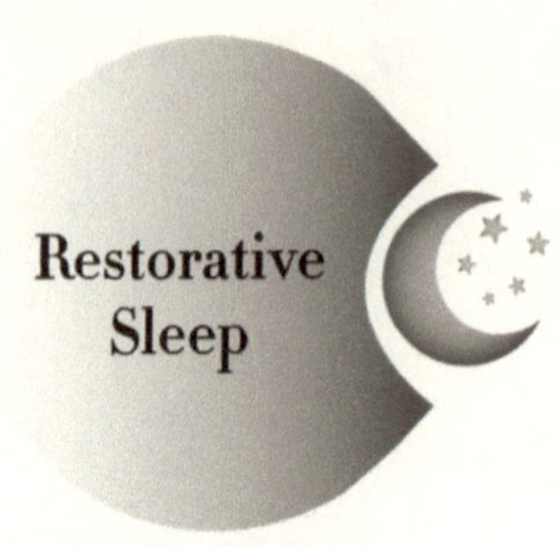

Restorative
Sleep

DEE-ism:

Go To The Dark Side.

You Need Your Sleep.

Restorative Sleep

Sleeping between 7 and 8 hours daily will allow your body to release HGH (Human Growth Hormones). The release of HGH slows the aging process, restores the body and repairs damage.

Applying the Senses

In a perfect world, where there is no shiftwork, no noisy neighbors, and only calm pets. True healthy sleep would be difficult to **see and hear** because its very existence, in its highest quality, would be in the darkest of dark and the quietest of quiet.

The **taste** associated with sleep might be toothpaste, and probably is, for most successful sleepers. Getting to the perfect sleep may **smell** like freshly dried laundry, or lavender, or the branded eucalyptus most of us know from childhood. To **touch** deep sleep might be to interrupt it, so precious is high-quality sleep. In a perfect world, it can **feel** like the ideal mattress, silk sheets, or flannel pajamas.

Go to http://deehealthnfitness.com/resources/ - password: 8xxx8 and check some of the guided meditation done by Rick Titan (ricktitan.com)

Defining Sleep

In this world—perfect or not—one thing is for certain. We all sleep. We all must sleep. Ever wonder why?

We all know when we don't get enough sleep we can't fully function the next day. After all, sleep deprivation is a torture technique—I know, let's not go there. It's also been proven in lab animals that, without sleep, there is certain disorientation and death—let's not go there either…well, not without a protest.

So, is sleep a protective mechanism? Well, just as hunger signals our body to eat—so we don't starve to death—tiredness is a sign that we need restorative time. It's a bonus that gravity, the sun, and the moon gift us, to help sync our body clocks to restorative bliss. *Shift worker alert: there are actions that can be taken to remedy unnatural patterns.*

How to Sleep Better

Getting a good night's sleep translates to using common sense. So, with sense(s) in mind, what does healthy sleep look, smell, and sound like? How does it feel to touch healthy sleep? Can we? Does healthy sleep have a taste?

Here's one you might not have heard before: Sleep Hygiene. Really, you ask? That's a thing? Yep, 'Sleep Hygiene' is a label that describes the ingredients of good sleep.

So, what can you do to have the cleanest sleeping habits? Do you anticipate a list of to-do's about to appear on the page? Are you already resisting in a 'what if I can't do them all' way? Are you all: 'Hey, Dee, I already feel pressure that you're going to ask me to make too many changes?'

Do I know you, or do I know you?

Relax. Read. This is the ultimate bedtime story.

Once Upon a Time There Was a Scary List—

1) Caffeine

2) Alcohol

3) Nicotine

4) Pain killers containing stimulants.

But, to fight against the scary list, there was a health advocate, named Dee, who wanted everyone to have pleasant dreams. She knew that the hot toddy recipe, from the internet, was a no-no. It may guarantee initial drowsiness, but then, after a few hours, would stimulate the brain and interrupt sleep.

This made Dee want to inform people about how important high-quality sleep is. She wanted people to experience restorative sleep.

Dee smiled about the phrase 'the sleeping environment.' She stressed to those she worked with that the sleeping environment just meant 'the place where a person has her bed.'

Dee promoted that the place where we sleep should be dark and cool. Like 'the bat-cave.' The temperature at night a cool 18-21degrees C (65 – 69 degrees F).

Dark, cool places are ideal for sleep. And it's a no brainer if there are city lights: black-out curtains. Black is always in style—light is a powerful cue for the brain to wake. Dee's list included: earplugs (if it's noisy). And no computer screens or electronics in the room.

"The light from our devices is 'short-wavelength-enriched,' meaning it has a higher concentration of blue light than natural light. And blue light affects levels of the sleep-inducing hormone melatonin more than any other wavelength." Scientific American

In all good stories there are animals. Dee told the animal household humans that if they were going to sleep with their pets, to think about whether the pet regularly woke in the night. If so, then maybe the pet would be better with its own cushion on the floor.

"The bedroom should be a sanctuary," said Dee, "with most of the square footage for sleep and intimacy. She asked her followers to eliminate clutter, and she reminded them that most mattresses wear out after ten years.

The people who knew and listened to Dee, felt that she made a lot of sense, and they believed they could do these things, even the declutter. They could always have an herbal tea instead of a coffee. A blanket would suffice (against the window) until they found some good drapes.

But then Dee added a twist to the plot. Something called a pre-bedtime routine.

Pre-Bedtime Ritual

The thing is, a pre-bedtime ritual is one of the most overlooked practices when finding a solution to sleeplessness. Nobody wants to invest in cutting the evening short. Everyone has worked too hard for that free time, right? I understand it is a big ask. People don't like to change too much.

But sleep starts before sleep. Prepping is necessary. It helps people rise earlier and fresher, so, in the end, it doesn't rob anyone of any time at all: it gifts time.

Ease the transition from wake time to sleep time with a period of relaxing activities an hour or so before bed. Stuff like taking a bath (the rise, then fall in body temperature promotes drowsiness). Other pre-bedtime prepping includes reading a book or practicing relaxation exercises.

Another must for a sleep-inducing environment is that there should be no stressful activities, no business-work, no emotional discussions. Physically and psychologically stressful activities can cause the body to secrete cortisol (the stress hormone). This only increases alertness. Repeat! The bedroom is for sleep and for intimacy only.

Rather than take their problems to bed, they could write those outstanding problems on a piece of paper, leave the paper out of the bedroom, and allow those things to be dealt with after sleep.

A piece of key advice: don't fight sleep, go with it. I love sleep and I want everyone to love it. I know it may take a while to get into some good sleep habits, but it will be so worth it.

Sometimes, I want to shout from the rooftops: "You have everything you need to begin to improve your sleep routine tonight. Need more free time? Sleep well. Looking for that ideal weight? Sleep well. Want to be in a better mood? Sleep well. Want to accomplish more? Sleep well.

And everyone who takes care of their sleep routine lived happily ever after, because good sleep means increased sex drive, enhanced creativity, and growth in productivity and efficiency.

Sleep Struggle Remedy

When you struggle to get a good, satisfying sleep, it can feel like there are many factors out of your control. This section is full of supportive tools to bring good sleep back into your wheelhouse.

To the dedicated shift workers out there - you are so appreciated. Emergency workers, flight crews, truckers, line-cooks, dishwashers, engineers, security guards:

You take the shifts that so many of us could not survive. Your work schedule makes it vital that you take extra care of your sleep and your health.

And to you night owls, reading this when most of us are asleep: I know those last hours of the day can be so rewarding and productive. But no matter how late your internal clock wants to keep you up, you still need at least 7-8 hours of quality sleep each night.

And to all of you who have other factors regularly impeding your sleep: I feel your pain and I have some remedies. You all deserve the best rest possible. Here's how the DEE-5 elements work together to help you achieve truly rejuvenating rest. My dear night owls, shift workers and sleep-deprived souls, this is especially important for you.

1) Movement and Exercise

Interrupted or shifting sleep patterns can mess with one's metabolism and hormones as well as be taxing to the immune system. Exercise and movement are keys to keeping the metabolism on track, and paramount to boost the immune system.

The best workouts for shift workers are High Intensity Interval Training (HIIT). HIIT is any workout session that alternates between intense bursts of activity followed by fixed periods of less intense activity, or even complete rest. (See exercise chapter for details.)

2) Food for Sleep

What you eat can either support or impede good sleep. Here are some guidelines for how to make sleep-supporting food choices:

- Limiting caffeine intake (under 400 milligrams a week (that's four cups).

- Avoiding all refined sugar. *I know, it's tough, but I value you and want you to be your healthiest selves.*

- Choosing organic and non-GMO foods— eating as naturally as possible. If it's in a box, it likely didn't just come out of the ground. If it spoils easily, it might actually be real food.

3) Soul-Work

Connecting to your deepest self and true stillness is a sleep-inducing bullseye. Try these options:

- Meditation is an incredible tool to reduce the level of stress that the body is going through due to the shift work or lack of sleep. Meditation and mindfulness is not woo-woo; it's a tool used by the most successful people, and totally supports high-quality sleep.

- Breathing exercises that allow being present, clean lungs, increase energy levels, and slow the heart rate, are helpful.

- Self-care practices such as being gentle with yourself, asking for help and being true to your own schedule.

In Real Life What Will You Do?

Here's How Bedtime Goes down at Our Place

My whole family is involved in the bedtime routine. Here's how my children and I do it:

- We ensure the last meal is 2-3 hours before bedtime. There is no caffeine consumed after dinner.

- Around 8:30 – 9ish we get ready for a tea: turmeric tea or chamomile with lavender. All members of the family participate.

- In this same time-block we put away all our electronics—they go on the counter in the kitchen.

- We each relax with our books and, in my case, I may journal about the successes of my day. I love finishing the day with positive thoughts.

This routine tells our bodies and minds that it is time to rest. No sleep issues in my house!

Recipe for Sleep

Turmeric Tea Golden Milk Recipe

Turmeric Tea or Golden Milk is a great way to get the benefits of turmeric daily. Enjoyed an hour or so before bed, it aids relaxation and helps boost the immune system while sleeping, and it's a natural anti-inflammatory.

Serves: 4

Ingredients

2 cups of milk of choice (almond, pecan, coconut, or dairy all work in this recipe)

1 teaspoon Turmeric

½ teaspoon Cinnamon

1 teaspoon raw honey or maple syrup or to taste (optional)

Pinch of black pepper (increases absorption)

Tiny piece of fresh, peeled ginger root or ¼ tsp ginger powder

Pinch of cayenne pepper (optional)

Instructions

Combine ingredients in a high-speed blender and smoothie it up.

Pour blended mix into a saucepan and heat for 3-5 minutes, over medium heat, until hot but not boiling.

Science Is Sexy. Sleep Is Sensual: Building on the 'Why' Of Sleep

Inactivity Theory

It's an old theory. Put simply: sleep served as a survival tool to keep some living beings out of trouble when they'd be the most vulnerable. Safe—to a point—while other living beings who were active at night poked around for food. The counter argument is that it is better to remain conscious. When one is awake and still, one can respond to an emergency. When one is sleeping…well, not so great.

So scientists moved on to another theory…that's what scientists do.

Energy Conservation Theory

The function of sleep reduces an individual's energy demand. Energy metabolism is significantly reduced during sleep (by as much as 10 percent in humans and even more in other species). Body temperature and caloric demand decrease during sleep. Did sleep evolve because we didn't always have food, so we had to conserve our energy?

Restorative Theory

The most powerful evidence that sleep serves to restore, repair, and rejuvenate is that animals, completely deprived of sleep, lose all immune function and die in a matter of weeks. This is further supported by findings that many of the major restorative functions in the body, like muscle growth, tissue repair, and growth hormone release occur mostly, or in some cases only, during sleep.

Here's some more mind-bending science: when we are awake, neurons called adenosine, build up in the brain. As long as we are awake, adenosine accumulates. At high levels we feel sleepy. (Scarily, caffeine can override the build-up.) During sleep, the body has a chance to clear adenosine, and as a result, we're more alert when we wake.

Brain Plasticity Theory

Sleep is correlated to changes in the structure and organization of the brain. It is clear, for example, that sleep plays a critical role in brain development of infants and young children. Babies sleep around fourteen hours out of every twenty-four, and about half that time is spent in REM sleep, the stage in which most dreams occur. A link between sleep and brain plasticity is becoming clear in adults as well, based on the effect that sleep (or sleep deprivation) has on our ability to learn and perform tasks.

Get Your Glow Back Theory

You know that moment when you fall exhausted into bed and your partner gives you the 'come hither' gesture or look? Are you often too tired to reciprocate their advances? It's entirely possible that being more consistently rested can bring your sexual appetite right back up to what's normal for you.

Lack of deeply restorative sleep can decrease the release of all your body's sex hormones. No sex hormones = lower or absent libido. On the other hand, when you are rested and energized, sex hormones are able to flow. You may also have more energy to play with your partner and explore creative sensuality which is so enriching for intimate relationships.

There is a common assumption that sex drive naturally decreases with age. Based on my experience as a Health and Fitness Coach, I don't believe this is a foregone conclusion. I believe that reduced libido at any age is a sign of potential imbalances in the body. In other words, you're not too old to have a good sex life, you're just not rested enough. With transformative sleep routines comes greater libido, more energy and motivation to sexually play, receive and give pleasure and, have the most romantic time with the person that you love most in this moment.

So, if you really want to bring the sensuality back into your life, sleep is the number one self-care item to commit to. Create a sleep routine and sleep the number of hours that your body needs (usually somewhere between 7-9 hours). After a consistent sleep routine, get ready for your glow to come back. Have fun with it!

*****

Q & A Time

"Dee, What about naps? To nap or not nap?"

If you're a nap person, great. But if you are finding it difficult to sleep at night, keep your naps short and before five o'clock if you're aiming for a 10:30 bedtime.

"Hey, Dee: I eat late. Will that affect my sleep?"

A wanna-be Buddhist walks into Pizza Hut and says: 'Make me one with everything."

If the 'one with everything' refers to a pizza rather than meditation then you're asking for trouble. A ten o'clock pizza delivery means insomnia for dessert. Keep nighttime eating light. It's better for your body, anyway, to eat more in the morning, less at lunch, and even less at dinner. Make sure you've eaten your final meal a few hours before bedtime. If you're hungry after that, snack on foods that (in your experience) won't disturb your sleep. Try making my tea recipe.

"Dear Dee, what about getting up and peeing in the night? I want to stay hydrated, but I don't want to keep running to the bathroom all night."

Drink enough fluid in the evening to keep from waking up thirsty, but not so much and so close to bedtime that you will be in the bathroom. If you do need to go to the washroom in the night, avoid the lights, keep those eyelids as sleepy as possible, and resist the urge to look at the clock. (Ideally the clock will be turned to the wall, and there will be no electronics in the bedroom.)

"Dee, does the time of day or night I exercise affect my sleep?"

Exercise helps promote restful sleep only if it is finished several hours before you go to bed. Exercise stimulates the body to secrete the stress hormone cortisol, which I've mentioned helps activate the alerting mechanism in the brain. This is fine, unless you're trying to fall asleep. Aim to finish exercising at least three hours before bed, or ideally, work out earlier in the day.

"Hi Dee, is there really an ideal time to go to bed? Someone told me that Eastern medicine says there is an exact time to sleep."

There are many studies, including those within Traditional Chinese Medicine, that recommend sleeping by 10:30pm since that's the time that the liver starts to repair, restore and cleanse itself. Whether it's 10:00pm or 11:00pm, the main thing is to keep things consistent. We have been programmed in Western culture that sleep is associated with being lazy. We are also consumers of time-filling activities that alter our internal clocks (video games, television). Bedtime should be a ritual that is revered and honored. Those who sleep well, perform well.

*****

Reader's Journal

How do I want my sleep to be?

What will I do to make that happen?

Currently, what does my sleep:
Look like:
Sound like:
Smell like:
Taste: like:
Feel like (touch):

What do I want my sleep to:
Look like:
Sound like:
Smell like:
Taste: like:
Feel like (touch):

I will check in next month to see if there are changes in what my sleep looks, sounds, smells, tastes, and feels like. (Put a date in your diary.)

What is the easy fix for me here?

What is the fix I'm shying away from?

(Hint, that's probably the one your mind-body-soul needs you to address.)

(Journal pages, recipes and resources available on the Happy Naked Exclusive Resources webpage http://deehealthnfitness.com/resources/ - password: 8xxx8

DEE-ism:

Food = Fuel Or Filler?

Applying the Senses

Supportive nutrition/healthy eating can **look** like a dramatic dance, a tango, perhaps. There is cooperation, steps and heat. It can appear as a partnership and partnering of leader and follower. Closer to the kitchen, supportive nutrition can **look** like a plate free of cracks, unchipped and squeaky clean, with a smooth texture. It can also take the shape of a bowl, a sacred vessel in which to place food that honors the body or a goblet in which to capture the bounty of a healthy elixir and the heavenly **scent** of its contents.

Healthy eating can **smell** like fresh fruit, raw carrots from the garden and, sometimes, a soup that has slowly simmered—all that bone broth vapor in the air. To **touch** healthy eating is to pluck an apple from a tree or feel dew-dropped blades of grass underfoot. It bubbles, it snaps, it hums, it crackles over a fire—the **sounds** of healthy eating. And we are left with **taste:** oh, the flavors. Sunny days. Outdoor swimming pools. Birthday parties in parks. Like swallowing celebration, itself. Like sipping on serendipity.

The Naked Truth about Nutrition

It has never been more important to be aware of the food we eat. That's because food sources are no longer the ones our ancestors harvested from. Chemically processed foods, use of pesticides, hormone and antibiotic treatments for animals are commonplace. Sugar added to create addictive tendencies—the forms of sugar are not natural: contrived molecular models, called sweeteners, fill many foods.

Our culture, formed around the practice of eating together, has evolved to eating on the run. Advertising has further altered our lifestyles by calling on us to supersize. The adage of 'more is better' is better for advertising giants and its food producing clients, than it is for the population at large. Media massively impacts our purchase, convincing us to 'experience bliss' by purchasing a 'tastes like real strawberries' pudding.

Pro-tip: Our bodies need to be nourished with 100% healthy food to optimally perform at all of life's stages.

Nutrition is the process of obtaining the food necessary for health and growth.

It's a branch of science. And, as we learned in the sleep section, science is sexy.

Food comprises a massive group of products. In a perfect world, that food is nutritional, promoting our health, growth and longevity.

Here's a little insight into why animals—let's not forget that's what we are—eat food:

1) As fuel, because it provides energy to help the body perform daily activities without feeling weak or sleepy.

2) To nurture the body and, in animal families/ packs, to share and socialize.

3) As a tool to heal, repair and restore the body.

In the world of socializing, no matter the culture, food and the practice of sharing meals sets emotional patterns.

Rarely do we think of food as fuel for our body, like premium gasoline for our cars. More often than not, about it as a reward, an indulgence, a break, in which to bury our tears and sadness, or the center of a social celebration.

By the time we are toddlers, our culture has impressed upon us what foods are 'good' and 'bad,' powerfully ingraining the role of food in our lives.

I can prove it with a little test. No, don't worry, this only requires a nanosecond.

Right now, think about your everyday eating. When you're ready, identify one food that you know is proven to be **unhealthy** for your body.

Ready. Set. Go!

A nanosecond was all you needed, right? Of course, you instantly knew 'one' thing. In that portion of one second, you probably thought of several and had to choose one. That's how deep-seated our *good* and *bad* cultural eating patterns are.

Your body, mind, and soul know instantly what is not healthy for you and that there's more than one of those things. Now we can touch on why you put something into your body that you know is not a 'healthy choice.'

How to Eat Better

Even though there are five areas I identify in living healthily, this part focuses on food and habits around food. Follow this section without the others and some parts of you will change. Dip into each of the DEE-5 System with eating as just one component of the whole journey to a sensual and spiritual you, and get ready to meet some interesting facets of yourself.

1) Mindful eating: eat at the table with family and zero technology or other distractions

2) Choose foods that are in season: visit local Farmers Markets, support local businesses

3) Choose food that is closer to the ground: fruits and vegetables mostly

4) Choose less processed food or eating out: practice home cooking or family cooking night

5) Drink water according to your weight and physical activity: Google water intake calculator to know the right amount for you

6) Clean up your pantry from junk, sugar or processed stuff: replace them with better options or an upgrade version

7) Communicate with your family about all these changes: take one step at the time and build on what you love to eat

In the journey of transforming your nutrition, take it slow and enjoy the feelings associated with lasting nourishment.

The Beautiful Synergy of Exercise and Nutrition

Eating well and regular exercise are like the twins in the Dee-5 family—closer to each other than to their siblings Healthy Sleep, Deep Spirituality and Mental Health. Like a lot of twins—exercise and nutrition work better as a pair. They feel each other's feels.

What do you think happens to your body when you lose weight without exercising?

When you lose weight without exercising your body will not be completely healthy. You may fool yourself into thinking it is because you feel 'happy' (that you got into a smaller size, that the scale says minus x, that someone questioned 'Have you lost weight?') but the weight you will lose will be lost without supporting muscle development. The weight loss will likely:

1) be regained easily and quickly

2) not be fat loss

3) not improve your inside-the-body health

4) prevent you from losing in the future, due to reduced metabolism

Weight is something we see on people—or not. Hence, 'You look great, have you lost weight?' Our insides are not visible to others. No one says, 'Hey, great arteries' or 'Wow, look at that clean gut, you must be pooping daily.'

Need confirmation? Take a typical runway model (extreme, I know). How do you think her heart health is?

Not developing muscle mass can be harmful to your body and unhealthy. Lack of movement, less muscle mass, and lack of balance and flexibility can paint your future with body aches and pain. Regular Exercise, that active twin of Eating Well, is paramount to your future and has direct positive effects on your eating.

Why We Do the Things We Do

Sometimes we eat or drink unhealthy stuff because of imbalanced hormones, high stress, or conditions that include cravings. Even when we decide to change our eating habits, the chemical patterns we've set in our body—or are predisposed to—can make it more challenging.

Many times, we eat or drink stuff that is not healthy for us out of a treat/reward mentality. An example of this is 'mommy and daddy are going out so here's some candy to eat with the babysitter.' 'Be a good girl and I'll bring you a treat.' 'Nice marks on that test, let's get you an ice cream'—an ice cream, over a childhood of treats becomes a sundae, becomes a banana split, becomes a regular occurrence of 'why not have this often?'

Diet Has Become a 4-Letter Word

The original meaning of the word 'diet' is a scientific description for the types of food we eat, but that has long been overshadowed and redefined to conjure images of weight loss and a steady stream of embattled 'losers' who feel exactly that: unworthy.

Commercial diets are really dreams for sale. Their price tag is high. The dreams are unrealistic scenarios and, many times, unhealthy too. Big business loves the word 'diet'—it's a multi-billion-dollar industry.

This is not a diet book. This is a love story. A manifesto of self-love. A lesson in how to engage all the senses when associating with food. Diet is currently a dangerous combination of four letters; it has lost its true original meaning. And has adopted a bottom-line commercial meaning of 'the program we go on (and off) to lose weight.'

Let's never use the word diet unless it has the original meaning, okay? If that is the only change you make, it is significant.

Inflammation

Most people in North America are suffering from inflammation of the body in different ways. This inflammation is recognized by joint pain, belly fat, fatty liver, bowel issues, and a number of other complaints. Whether it is known or not, we can reduce inflammation by eliminating or reducing foods we know are responsible for inflammation.

The top inflammatory foods are:

1) Red meat

2) Alcohol

3) Dairy

4) Gluten

5) Sugar

6) Processed food, including junk food

For those of us who eat animal protein such as red meat, chicken, pork, eggs and fish, it is strongly recommended to source organic, grass fed animals, free of artificial hormones and antibiotics.

NOTE ON HORMONES

For men who eat chicken as their source of protein: it is important to be educated on the source of the chicken to avoid what are called 'man boobs' caused from ingesting an excess of female hormones which are present in chickens that have been fed hormones to increase the breast meat.

Canada is exceptionally responsible when it comes to organic food. However, much of the organic food on our shelves is from the USA. The FDA regulations are not the same in the USA as Canada's stricter guidelines for qualification and certification. Caution is always advised when sourcing organic food imported from another country.

As well as checking the authenticity of food sources, it is essential to double check information. The internet is rampant with sales pitches and quotes that simply link to the blogposts of others; not necessarily an original, highly qualified, ethically minded publication. Click responsibly. Read, and verify the roots of the information.

www.agr.gc.ca

www.canada.ca/en/health-canada

Choose local food to support local growth businesses and economy.

As a Canadian consumer located in western Canada, I source my produce food from SPUD.ca. SPUD provides more details than the grocery store, including exactly where the food comes from. Check them out.

Your local organic store stocks foods that are dense in nutritional value. Many are familiar in name, and others may be new to you. They are called Super Foods. Check out:

- goji berries

- chamomile - the flower itself

- lavender flower

- bee pollen/ royal honey

- cacao nibs

Balance Instead Of Portion

When we eat healthy food there is little need for stringent portion control. Our bodies let us know when they are full as we get used to fueling with healthy foods. The ideal plate—regardless of the amount of healthy food on the plate—is as follows:

50%-80% of healthy carbs

25%-35% of clean and healthy protein

10% healthy fat

Can't picture it? Think of your favourite round plate. Divide it into two. Fill one half and some more with healthy carbs. Take the remaining piece and add some clean protein. Take a final sliver and make that a healthy fat.

Two brilliant and informative documentaries, available on Netflix, about food selection, source, and sensibility are: *Fat, Sick and nearly Dead* - by Joe Cross;

Cooked – by Michael Pollan.

So, what foods are in the healthy list? What will be on your plate?

Healthy Carbs

Vegetables

Legumes/Beans

Fruits

Healthy Proteins

Legumes/Beans (also carb)

Avocado (also fat)

Broccoli (yes, really)

Grass fed red meat, pork, and chicken

Free range fish (to avoid ingesting mercury)

Healthy Fats

Coconut oil

Avocado (also protein)

Seeds and nuts (also protein)

By combining healthy carbs, protein and fat at each meal there is no need to worry about portions, since all simple carbs (bread, pasta, white rice, gluten, processed foods, and fast/junk foods) are not on that plate.

Dee's Dirty Dozen

Reduce or eliminate these from your kitchen to get an instant boost to your health.

- Ketchup, mustard, mayonnaise

- Non-organic red meat, pork, fish, and chicken

- Margarine

- All processed fruit juices

- Soft drinks/soda pop

- Cow's milk

- Yogurt

- Most cheeses

- Processed meats such as ham and sausage

- White and brown sugar

- Desserts including ice cream and cake

- Chips, microwave popcorn, flavoured blends of nuts/commercial 'trail and snack mixes'

*****

In Real Life What Will You Do?

Here's how 'Healthy Belly' Goes Down In Our House

- We cook once a week for the whole week.

- Sometimes we cook even more than a week's worth and freeze.

- We enjoy beans in a lot of our recipes.

- We eat a lot of quinoa. We eat it as a side dish, in our salad, with spinach, corn (Non-GMO), tomato, onion, broccoli, and cauliflower; anything really — the sky's the limit. Add real lemon juice. Put this salad in the fridge and grab a bowl anytime.

- We love soups.

- We eat cooked chicken, red meat (grass fed) and fresh fish.

- We make lots of brown rice and include it in various dishes.

- Pre-chopping foods like pineapple, watermelon, melon is a timesaver.

- We always clean all our veggies and fruits as soon as we get in from grocery shopping. We use apple cider vinegar and baking soda for cleaning our veggies and fruit.

- Everything is cleaned before it goes into the fridge. (Believe it, it becomes habit. And once you're used to it, when someone brings something into your home you'll wonder if it has been cleaned.)

- We enjoy online grocery shopping using services like SPUD.ca. It has been a great time saver. I like the quality, plus one delivery van going to several homes helps the planet too. (If you are in Alberta or British Columbia - Canada, and want to register, use this referral code: CAL-MAGDEN to get a discount on your order.)

- If the budget allows, we buy large quantities of items that store well.

Planning ahead is an excellent way for our busy family to move from event to event. We always pack school lunches the night before. Something else we do at night is to leave oatmeal overnight with water, then add seeds and nuts and fruit in the morning. It's great warmed up or cold.

This Is How It Might Feel When You Make The Shifts

When you begin changing grocery shopping and eating habits you might feel lost since a lot of things will be eliminated that are related to:

Your culture

Your family

Your own customs; the only things you know

I will share a few strategies to make your life easier, especially when you have kids, a full-time job, a spouse in your busy life. But also know, *there is no busy, just different priorities.*

In case you're already waiting to ask about some of your favorites and you're already in withdrawal thinking you have to eliminate something completely: no one has said you can never have foods that your culture enjoys, or that you have associated with something 'fun,' be it popcorn at the movies, and

IKEA hot dogs, or a Snickers Bar. The thing is, you will only truly enjoy those foods when you do not crave them. When they don't have power over you. When they are a choice. As you change your choices to natural foods, the cravings for fast foods of poor quality will subside.

*****

Easy Meals That Can Create Sustainable Habits

DEE-ism:

Breakfast As A Warrior.

Lunch As A Goddess.

Supper As A Light-Filled Spirit

Aim for three meals with three snacks in between. Basically, eat six times a day. That is basically every 2-3 hours.

Breakfast

I am a huge advocate of having breakfast. It powers the body for the day. It supports all the work the body did during the night.

When people ask my opinion on morning protein shakes, I have to say that I am all about eating food that is as close to the ground as possible. A protein shake is like taking a chicken and making it into powder—you can get all the benefits by eating the chicken in its natural form.

Another thing about protein shakes is that protein is not the first source of energy you need for your day. The first fuel you need is carbs. Of course, always consider that every meal needs to be balanced.

Oatmeal with fruits, nuts, and seeds. No need to add any honey since the fruits will add the sweetness.

Smoothies: 80% veggies and 20% fruits—could add a little honey—add nuts and seeds. Want more variety? Add avocado or coconut oil for fat.

Plate some veggies: spinach, beets, carrots, broccoli, cucumber, cooked sweet potato, choose a couple.

Enjoy some fruits: banana, apples, grapes, choose a couple.

Invent a 'Power Sandwich' with a whole grain bread or gluten free, and stuff it with lettuce and/or spinach; tomato, onion, alfalfa and avocado; cheese and ham if you wish. Add an egg to that sandwich if you like.

Lunch

Lunch should fuel your body to power you through the afternoon. If you feel bloated or heavy after your meal, there was something that your stomach could not process. It is a sign that it is taking all your energy to digest instead of energizing you.

Pay attention to your body because it might be telling you things and sending you signals of food that you should not be eating.

Go for, salad with beans or animal protein and avocado.

Add nuts and seeds to that salad.

Dress it with real lemon juice or lime.

Make a lettuce wrap. Fill with veggies and a protein and be sure to pop in some avocado.

Create a crazy quinoa salad by taking all the 'healthy foods' you have available, including beans, and dress it with lemon or lime juice.

Stir up a pot of legume soup with sweet potato, onion, pepper, squash or vegetable/chicken/or meat broth. If you make bone broth, that is an excellent alternative.

Dinner

In North American culture, supper is the heaviest meal of the day. But, since the body is getting ready to sleep, it is better to eat something light and easy to digest. At this time of day, the body doesn't need a lot of energy.

Supper is an excellent meal for protein. This is because this protein will help repair and restore all the tissue damaged by doing the regular activities through the day.

Keep the portion small and remember to eat 2-3 hours before going to sleep. In this case, your body will do what it is supposed to do: restore itself instead of processing the food you had for supper.

A great dinner for kids is cereal and almond milk. An egg goes down nicely with that.

Smoothie with lots of greens instead of colorful veggies.

Small plate of beans or quinoa salad.

An omelet with veggies.

Small bowl of soup with some nuts on the side.

Snacks

Snacks are something to fill your day between the big meals. We are looking at eating every 2 to 3 hours and a total of 5 to 6 meals a day.

Grab a small handful of almonds.

Homemade granola bars (regular granola bars have a lot of sugar, fructose, corn syrup).

Take a smaller portion of lunch, breakfast, or supper.

Eat whole fruits.

Snag a cup of a previously made smoothie.

Pop some carrots and cucumber in a bag.

Enjoy a serving of roasted chickpeas.

A Favorite Snack Recipe – Power Balls

Ingredients

½ cup (raw) cashews

1 cup medjool dates, pitted

2 Tablespoons cocoa powder (organic or fair trade)

½ cup raw peanut butter or raw almond butter

⅓ cup Raw honey

¼ cup ground flaxseed

⅛ teaspoon sea-salt (optional)

2 tablespoon chia seeds

⅓ cup (raw) sunflower seeds

¼ cup almond flour or almond meal or cashew/ almond crushed (for coating)

Preparation

1) Grind the nuts, set aside. (Do not pulverize).

2) Blend the dates.

3) Put dates into a bowl and add cocoa. Use your hands to work it in.

4) Add peanut butter and honey and continue mixing.

5) Add cashews, flaxseed, sea-salt chia, and sunflower.

6) Knead until combined.

7) Roll mixture into one-inch balls.

8) Roll each in almond meal and set aside.

9) Enjoy or store in fridge for up to ten days.

Smart Shopping

In the interest of saving money and being a conscientious shopper, when you buy the following items note that you do not have to purchase all organic. See the list below. The Dirty Dozen focuses on foods that should be purchased in organic form. The clean fifteen are not foods that have to be purchased in organic form—you can still get good value and nutrition from those items in their commercial form.

The Dirty Dozen and Clean Fifteen have been publicized by the EWG – The Environmental Working Group. Its tireless efforts have helped and continue to make the planet a better place. www.ewg.org.

So here they are, for your shopping smarts and carts:

CLEAN FIFTEEN™: don't be over-concerned if you cannot find organic avocados, corn, pineapples, cabbage, sweet peas, onions, asparagus, mangos, papayas, kiwi, eggplant, honeydew, grapefruit, cantaloupe, cauliflower. These are the clean fifteen.

DIRTY DOZEN™: if you are buying the following, please buy organic: strawberries, apples, nectarines, peaches, grapes, cherries, celery, spinach, tomatoes, cherry tomatoes, bell peppers, cucumbers. These are the dirty dozen.

Wait! I'm not done. Will I ever shut up? Well, you've probably seen my videos. I care about everyone. I'm unapologetically passionate.

Nutritional Supplements

There are a lot of things that you can do to supplement and get more nutrients into your body.

Probiotics can restore your intestinal balance. If you purchase a probiotic in capsule, powder, or liquid form, ensure it has at least 10 billion active cells per 'capsule' (or serving).

One way to introduce probiotics into your life is by fermenting. Making your own fermented food can be simple as well. Head online to find some awesome recipes that require hardly any effort.

Omega 3, found in flaxseed, is another excellent supplement. Be sure to make sure it has an elevated number of EDP (1000mg), not only fish oil.

Essential oils are an amazing addition to helping your body function. For example, peppermint oil to help your digestive system.

*****

Questions from Clients

"Holy crap, Dee. What the heck should I put in my cart then? I'll never stick to this diet." Failed Before I Try.

Dear FBIT, let me start by repeating: it's not a diet. We need to be careful in using the word diet. What I'm suggesting is choosing foods that fuel the body. It's change for sure. Yet, it's a return to how we were meant to eat. It's respecting our bodies.

So, here's an idea. Put these things in the list below into your cart, then have fun. Don't be scared of them. Did you know that most people eat the same ten foods and just prepare them in different ways? Spice it up, change it up, health it up. Don't worry about portion sizes. Think balance, think fuel, think new, adventure, real, pure, energy. If your mind wanders to the word 'diet', stop. If you find yourself telling a friend you're on a 'diet', stop.

Lettuce

Spinach

Onion (real one, not powder)

Tomato

Garlic (real, not powder)

Carrots (no baby carrots, the real size)

Mushrooms

Bok choy

Ginger (always the root, not the powder)

Turmeric (root and powder depends on the season)

All sorts of fruits

Potato and sweet potato

Beets

Alfalfa (germinated)

Sweet pepper

Cabbage

Celery

Cilantro, parsley

Quinoa

Quinoa pasta – gluten free

Beans: lentils, black beans, split peas, chickpeas

Brown rice – gluten free

Oregano, Himalayan salt (or sea salt), black pepper

Apple cider vinegar and soy sauce (brand name: BRAGG)

Cereal (brand name: Nature's Path)

Oatmeal (organic)

Almond milk or coconut milk, Non-GMO. (*Making your own is super-fast, cheaper, has NO preservatives, or sugar, and can be made in small batches. It's amazing.*)

Gluten free bread, or whole wheat, or organic sourdough

Cheese (chose the one with less and simple ingredients) goat is good.

Organic coffee, green tea, chamomile tea, lavender tea, night tea, or a variety of herbal teas.

"Dee, okay, I'm embarrassed. I don't know what GMO is. I hear the name Monsanto, but I don't know what GMO means." –Uninformed

Hey, we can't know everything. There's no need to be embarrassed. Kudos to you for asking. It shows you're interested. It's a great question, and guess what? I've been asked it before. You're not the only one.

GMO stands for Genetically Modified Organisms. Sometimes called GM's. They are also called Genetically Engineered Foods or Bioengineered Foods. This means they are foods which are produced from organisms that have had changes introduced into their genetic structure (their DNA). This brings about new, selected traits in the food. The genetic changes are treated differently (in some cases) by the human digestive system. In other words, they are not natural foods, even if they claim to be filled with nutrition.

GMOs are controversial because of their impact on the environment and impact on the food chain.

"Dee, how do I know if something is a processed food?" - Janis

Janis: It's fairly basic. The thing that has made identifying processed food difficult is packaging, it uses language and color that tricks us into believing it is natural. Well, here's the rub: usually, like almost all the time, if it's packaged its processed. So, it's time to think outside the box, the jar, the can, the tetra pack.

Ask yourself any of these questions when you are considering a food.

Has it been changed from its original form?

Did it ever have an original form?

Does it have additives: sugars and chemicals?

*****

Reader's Journal

91

How do I want my grocery shopping experience to:
Look:
Smell:
Sound:
Taste:
Feel:
How do I want the inside of my fridge to:
Look:
Smell:
Sound:
Taste:
Feel:

What will I do to make that happen?

Currently, what does my eating?
Look like:
Sound like:
Smell like:
Taste: like:
Feel like (touch):

What do I want my eating?
Look like:
Sound like:
Smell like:
Taste: like:
Feel like (touch):

I will check in next month and see if there are changes in what my food choices, taste, smell, feel, sound, look like. How has my kitchen evolved in terms of all the senses?

What are three things I can do right now that will not cause me grief?

(Example, clean out my cupboards so the foods I don't need are not on display.)

What is the thing about eating that I'm fighting/that scares me the most?

(Example, I won't be able to go out with the girls for wing night.)

What have I never tried from the food list in this section?

Make your own grocery list here (and carry it with you):

Always do a monthly review. It's good to get a view of the big picture. After all, small changes, over time, make lasting impact.

Find a handy downloadable journal page, food journal and grocery list on the Happy Naked Exclusive Resources http://deehealthnfitness.com/resources/ - password: 8xxx8

Complete Excercise

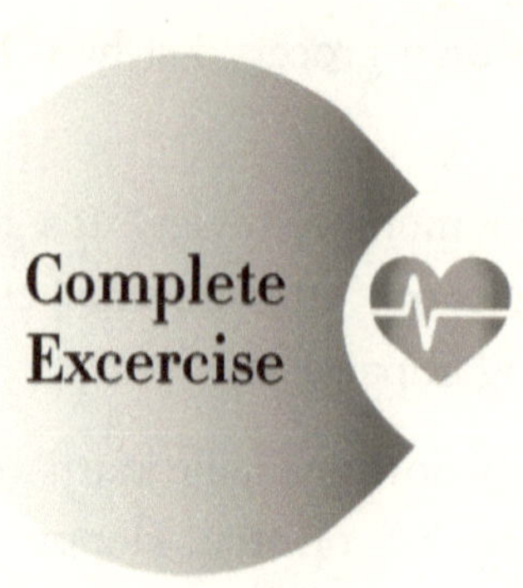

DEE-ism:

Pound the Pavement Like You're Playing
the Drums.

Dance to The Rhythm of Feeling Good Naked.

Applying the Senses

Sometimes complete exercise **smells** like clean socks from the washing line, that kind of freshness. Complete exercise's flavor may cry out to be a green smoothie, but more often it **tastes** like a tall glass of water, even lime and soda, served with a thick slice of blue sky. It **appears** as a kite flying, that tail so free, the mood so happy. To **touch** complete exercise is to hold a terry-towel bath sheet after a long shower. It also feels to the fingers like a smooth, heavy, bowling ball releasing from the hand and resulting in a strike. Complete exercise, in essence, a healthy body, **sounds** like laughter after a gutter ball, cheering after a strike, and the rhythm of one's own footsteps as they walk, hike, jog, run and/or step in joy.

As I see it, our physical bodies are ultimately:

A tool.

A vehicle.

Equipment to perform activities.

The most perfect creation.

The human body is so perfect that it has the ability and capacity to restore and repair itself, as long as it is provided with the right fuel to do so and has the right daily maintenance: movement, thoughts and sleep.

Everyone has a unique body: different height, weight, bone size, muscle mass. According to our genes we also have the capacity to further develop that body.

There are three rules that I ask everyone I work with to absorb and make their own. *One of three-I am me. Two of three-take time to see. Three of three-kind and free.*

One of Three - I Am Me

I will not build and shape my body like you; you will not build and shape your body like me.

Engaging in self-care through fuel, exercise, sleep quality, mental health, and spiritual enlightenment, is not a body, mind and soul competition. It is an opportunity for individual life-enhancing body fulfillment and contentment.

When it comes to food and exercise: your body is unique, and as long as you provide the right fuel (food) and the right maintenance (exercise), your body will thank you by shaping you as you were naturally intended.

Your body is powerful: as you start and continue physical activities, as well as challenge yourself to advance, your body will adapt. It will perform for you.

I believe that by shaping your body through fuel and movement, your soul and spirit will take on a wondrous journey. As you feel more confident in taking part in physical activity, as you become more comfortable in your physical self, a level of internal contentment will manifest.

I see exercise as a process of transformation from outside-in. Some people use personal growth, energy work, meditation, or yoga to transform; exercise is another tool which is just as beneficial.

Two of Three - Take Time to See

PLEASE give yourself enough time to refresh, renew, and reshape your body. This is not a race. It's not a short-term plan. It is a lifestyle, a forever shift.

Please allow your body to get used to the changes. Do not look for short-term results. Three months will show a difference, four to twelve months will provide more evidence, but from day one, there will be a chemical change from your decision making with that first movement.

Why This Much Time to See Real Results?

Many people have been developing different diseases and conditions over time. Many have built up huge amounts of stress and they suffer from various aches and pains. Most of my clients have not been in touch with their bodies for five to ten years.

Ten years? That's a decade of mistreatment—back, heel, ankle pain, blood pressure issues, diabetes, high cholesterol, inflammation, belly fat, weight gain (that is, categorized as overweight, obese, or having belly fat). Give yourself enough time for your body to heal and adjust to the new way of living.

In this process of transformation there will be relapses. That's okay; we are all human. We learn from relapse. Sometimes there are times of feeling lost. This is where I step in—through this book—to help you with your DETERMINATION. I want to assist you on the journey to feeling extraordinary.

Three of Three - Kind And Free

BE KIND with yourself.

This is a journey for life—your Life. Some days you will feel like not exercising and other days you will feel like running a marathon. It is a step by step process of getting used to and adapting to this new lifestyle.

Because this is a process, I suggest scheduling workouts from 5 minutes to 30 minutes. The reason is that excuses are not an option not to work out. Having scheduled workouts means they will be checked off, just like brushing your teeth. Being active and healthy is your NUMBER ONE PRIORITY since your body is the only vehicle you have been given in this lifetime.

My Journey from Frustration to Transformation

For many years, I set only short-term goals, four weeks was a common duration for me. I wanted to see results like less belly fat and more tone in my butt, legs, and arms. I started jogging and doing more weights and elastics. Of course, I did not see the results I wanted because four weeks is not a long time. And, capital L-Life happens. Three kids, married, then separated, a full-time job and a hectic social life. Lots of upheaval, busy-ness and change.

Then, a year later, a friend of mine suggested I commit to a 60-day program. No excuses. And so, my friend, my brother and I did six days a week for eight weeks —no excuses. None.

What happened? I saw results. I felt incredible, agile and motivated to keep going. Then life happened again.

I realized that it wasn't about 4 weeks, 8 weeks, or a 30-day challenge, it was about a lifestyle change without being negatively—dysfunctionally—tied to a calendar. Ultimately, every day mattered.

I decided to shape my body every single day of my life. I used a calendar so I could say, 'what would this be like for one year?' I took a year to create new lifestyle habits.

I took a picture of myself in the summer of 2013, saved it somewhere, then forgot about it. I set about changing my eating habits and exercising as many days of the weeks as possible—WITHOUT EXCUSES. I always made sure that exercise was part of my daily routine; some days five minutes, some days sixty minutes—it probably averaged thirty minutes a day.

In the summer of 2014, I remembered taking the picture the previous summer. I took another picture and then pulled out the year-old one. Side by side. Wow. Making a lifestyle change rather than a short-term goal had made all the difference.

I learned to be kind with myself. I learned how have reasonable and realistic expectations of myself each and every day. I gave myself moments of grace when I could just *be*. Just *be* a mom or just *be* an entrepreneur. Or just *be* Dee sitting quietly connecting to myself.

Fast forward to 2018. I had fully accepted the fact that, having my own business, kids and life, it's vital that I am realistic with my goals and creative in implementing my daily workout to align with the fact that my body is also aging. I believe that we can be, like wine 'better with age.'

Life doesn't have to be all about rules, but I did come up with three main ones for me—that I have shared with you—so there is some structure to changing your life and avoiding as much frustration as possible.

Why Exercise?

It is the only tool we have—in our current era—to keep the physical body healthy, because:

- We don't hunt for food like our ancestors did.

- We don't move as much as other generations, we drive to go to places.

- Many of us spend 8 -11 hours a day seated.

- Canada's winters can be harsh. Most people have little or no inclination to do outdoor activities.

Exercise is scientifically proven to:

- Keep your vehicle in top shape, by increasing and then maintaining your muscle mass, flexibility and balance, naturally lost as we age.

- Release more HGH (Human Growth Hormone) and slow the aging process.

- Boost levels of energy. More energy, better performance.

- Support healthy sleep. Healthy sleep allows regeneration of body and brain.

- Help avoid injury and promote healing when we do incur problems—mental and physical.

Big Intentions, Sporadic Participation, False Starts

Most people who want to lose weight and/or feel more active do exactly this:

1) Get a GYM Membership.

2) Tell their friends they got a gym membership.

3) Buy some workout clothes to wear at the gym.

That is what they do.

Rarely do they go.

And if they do go, they may not have been to one before. Being in this situation can be very intimidating. For those who actually get to the gym, their first choice is the treadmill or stationary bike. Why? Because it's pretty much two things we all know how to do: walk and ride a bike.

Don't want to throw your money away and still not exercise? Here's how:

Save your money.

Start at home.

This is doable. Un-intimidating. Little or no equipment needed. And it will yield results.

Get Used To Moving – Easy Start

The workout below is designed to be done two days a week for 90 days. Within the 90 days, people begin to develop the habit of exercising consistently. When you're ready, add an extra day of exercise each week. By the time you require more challenge, the sets can be increased from 3 to 5, or more.

To boost your overall activity level, you can also compliment other forms of exercise and movement that you may already do. Common examples are walking, climbing stairs, playing with children and gardening.

Take notes after each workout; it is vital to track your results, taking into consideration:

How tired you feel after or mid workout.

How you feel at the end of the workout.

How many reps or sets you can do before feeling exhausted.

Whether you feel that it is not challenging enough, or way too challenging.

If you have the need to add weights or more resistance.

There are lots of workout tracking sheets and resources on the *Happy Naked Exclusive Readers' Resource* webpage.

Specific to this workout, think about three steps or levels. It can be a lower intensity warm-up with emphasis on using the exercises as stretching/getting ready, an absolute beginner's primer in which the routine is modified (see modifications with graphics), or a basic workout. In fact, the entire series could be all three in one session. 1) A warm-up at low intensity. 2) The workout. 3) A return to low intensity to transition out of a complete workout.

That's the beauty of this routine: it bends itself around your needs.

Example of modification for warm-up or absolute beginners—the jumping jack, do it without jumping (simply do a flying action—be the bird).

This workout is designed for beginners or could be a warm-up for a person who is advanced in their fitness level. Full instructions including photos for each exercise follow the workout schedule pages.

Workout – Week # 1 - Day #1

High Knees – 20 reps

Squats – 15 reps

Push ups – 5

Plank – 10 seconds

Workout – Week # 1 - Day # 2

Jumping Jacks – 20 reps

Lunges – 30 reps (15 each leg)

Mountain Climber – 30 reps in total

Superman – 10 seconds

Workout – Week # 2 - Day #1

High Knees – (20 reps) x 2 Sets

Squats – (15 reps) x 2 sets

Push ups – (5 Reps) x 2 sets

Plank – 20 seconds

Workout – Week # 2 - Day # 2

Jumping Jacks – (20 reps) x 2 sets

Lunges – (30 reps (15 each leg)) x 3 sets

Mountain Climber – (30 reps in total) x 2 Sets

Superman – 20 seconds

Workout – Week # 3 - Day # 1

High Knees – (20 reps) x 3 Sets

Squats – (15 reps) x 3 sets

Push ups – (5 Reps) x 3 sets

Plank – 30 seconds

Workout – Week # 3 - Day # 2

Jumping Jacks – (20 reps) x 3 sets

Lunges – (30 reps (15 each leg)) x 3 sets

Mountain Climber – (30 reps in total) x 3 Sets

Superman – 30 seconds

Increase sets until you get to five sets for each exercise. Complete 6 weeks and journal your progress and successes.

Here Are the Exercises

High-Knee

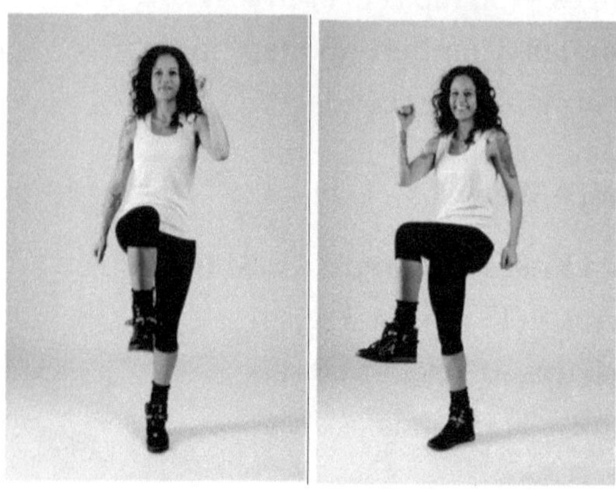

Stand straight, feet should be a hip width apart, look straight ahead, arms hanging by your side. Jump from one foot to the other while lifting your knee as high as possible, hip height advisable. Arms should be following the motion. Touch the ground with the balls of your feet.

Squat

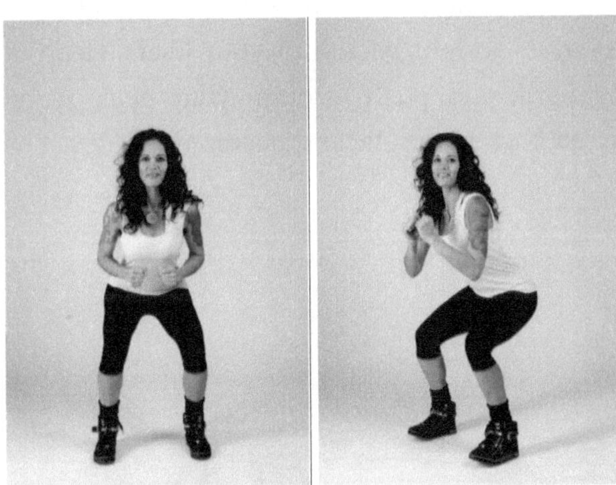

Stand with your head facing forward and your chest held up and out. Place your feet shoulder-width apart or slightly wider. Extend your hands straight out in front of you to help keep your balance. You can also bend the elbows or clasp the fingers.

Sit back and down like you're going to sit in an imaginary chair. Keep your head facing forward as your upper body bends forward a bit. Rather than allowing your back to round, let your lower back arch inward slightly as you descend.

Lower yourself so your thighs are as parallel to the floor as possible, with your knees over your ankles. Press your weight back into your heels. Keep your body tight, and push through your heels to bring yourself back to the starting position.

Push-Up

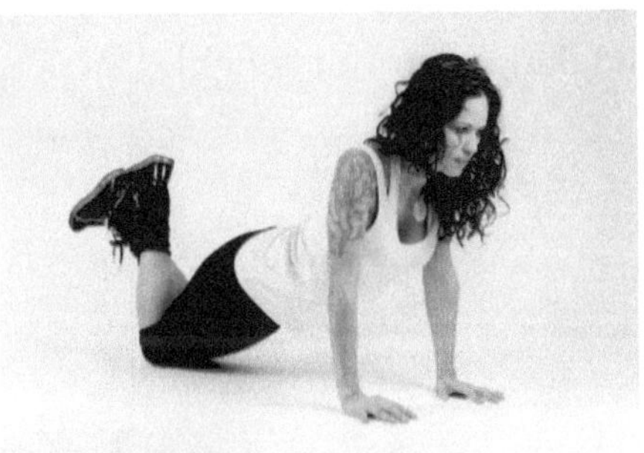

Get into a high plank or knee position. Place your hands firmly on the ground, directly under shoulders. Begin to lower your body—keeping your back flat and eyes focused about three feet in front of you (parallel with the rest of the body) to keep a neutral neck—until your chest grazes the floor.

Push back up.

Modification: If you do not feel ready to go with a full-body push-up, like in this picture, then there are two options.

1) Lower the knees and push up from having the knees on the floor.

2) Even gentler: use the counter or dinner table and push from that height. This way you're inclined, but not taking your full weight.

Plank

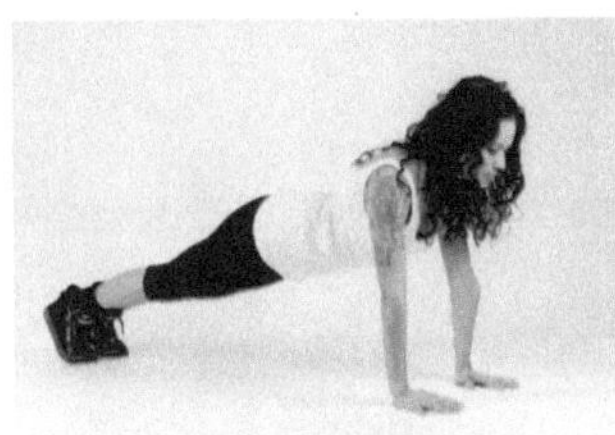 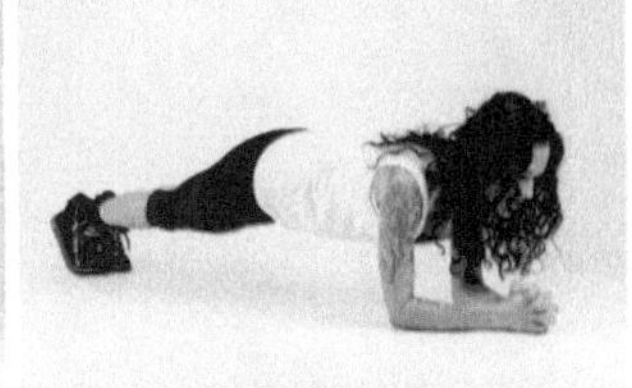

High Plank 1   Low Plank 2

Start by getting into a press up position. Bend your elbows and rest your weight on your forearms (2) or on your hands. (1)

Your body should form a straight line from shoulders to ankles.

Engage your core by sucking your belly button into your spine.

Hold this position for the prescribed time.

Modification for beginners: add a bit of inclination — a countertop, a table, or 'whatever is not the floor.'

Jumping Jack

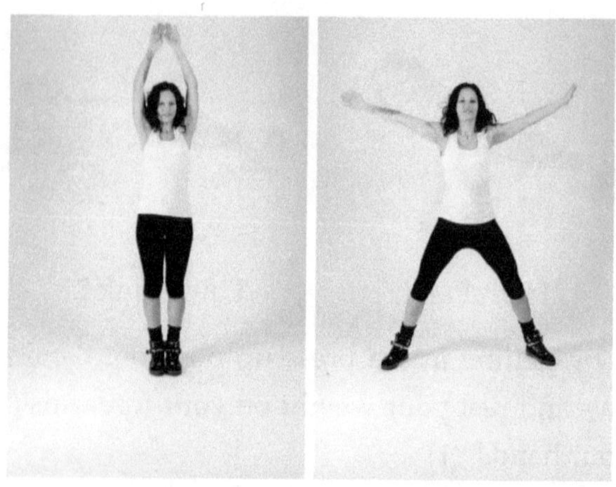

Stand with feet together, knees slightly bent, and arms to sides. Jump while raising arms and separating legs to sides. Land on forefoot with legs apart and arms overhead. Jump again while lowering arms and returning legs to midline.

Modification – no jumping.

Simply create the motion and move legs from side to side.

Or, narrow your stance and squat while doing the arms.

Or, raise knees each side while doing the arms.

Lunges

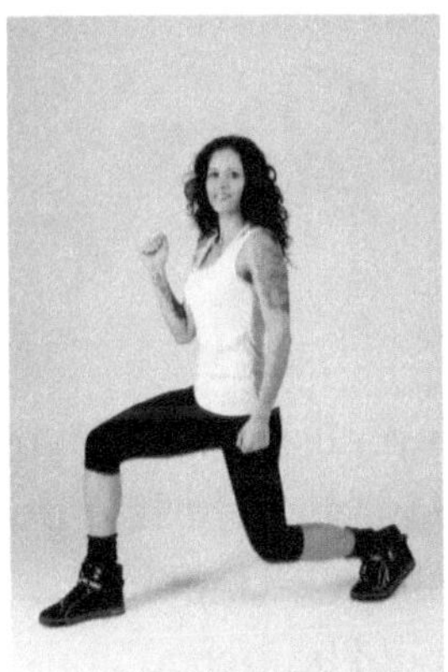

Keep your upper body straight, with your shoulders back and relaxed and chin up (stare at a chosen point in front so you are not tempted to look down). Always engage your core.

Step forward with one leg, lowering your hips until both knees are bent at about a 90-degree angle.

Modification for beginner lunges: remain stationary —don't step forward—just switch legs. When you have more control, you can raise your arms as is done in the complete exercise (illustrated).

Want more of a challenge? Step backward instead of stepping forward.

Mountain Climber

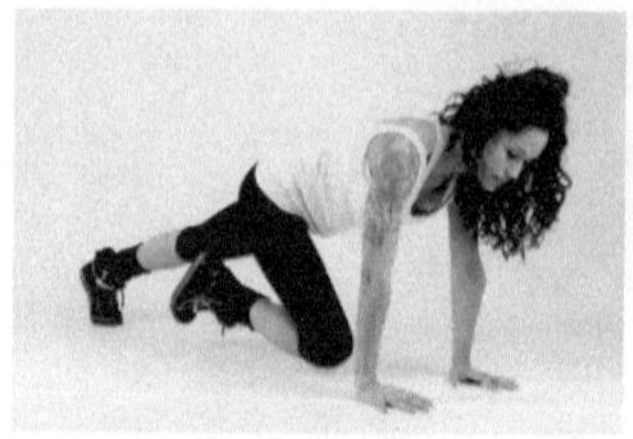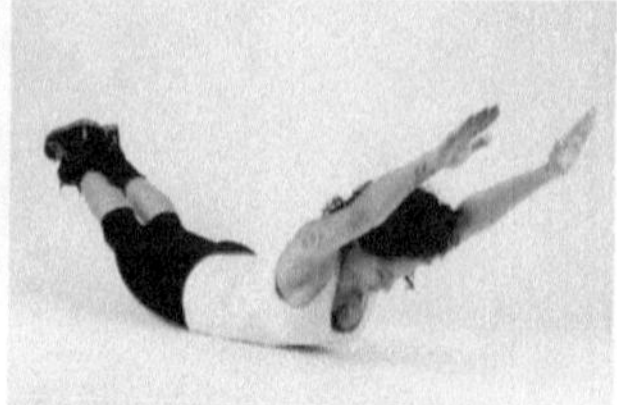

Assume a push-up position with your arms straight and your body in a straight line from your head to your ankles. Without changing the posture of your lower back (it should be arched), raise your right knee toward your chest.

Pause, return to the starting position and repeat with your left leg. That's one rep. Alternate until you've completed all your reps.

Modification: go to countertop and bring knees close to chest in a kind of 'high-knee' so that it's less of a lean and more of a high-knee march (while leaning against the countertop).

Superman

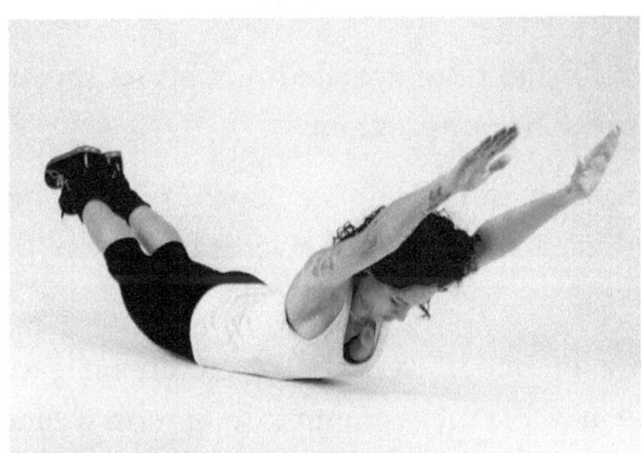

Lie straight and face down on the floor or exercise mat. Your arms should be fully extended in front of you.

Simultaneously raise your arms, legs, and chest off the floor and hold this contraction for 2 seconds.

Tip: Squeeze your lower back to get the best results from this exercise. Remember to exhale during this movement.

Note: When holding the contracted position, you should look like Superman when he is flying.

Slowly begin to lower your arms, legs and chest back down to the starting position while inhaling.

Repeat for the recommended number of repetitions prescribed in your program.

Modification: can't lie on the floor? Try standing - do everything above, but from a vertical position (feet on the floor).

I'm big on modifications. By modifying exercise, people find that they commit to long-term wellness—basically no one is overwhelmed to begin. And, there is a sense of success. I'd be thrilled to go through modifications with you personally.

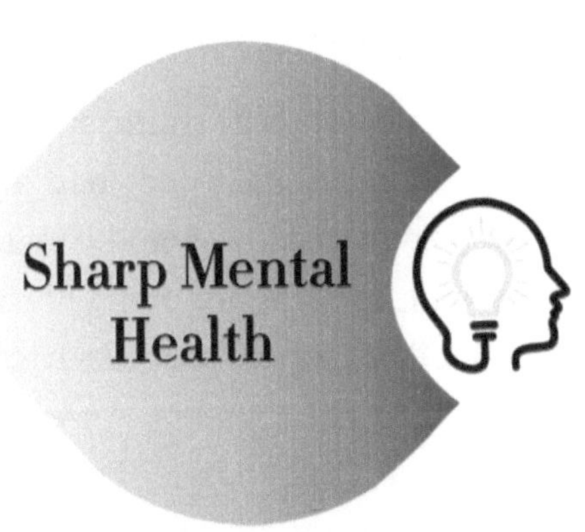

Sharp Mental Health

DEE-ism:

TRUST in your SELF

CELEBRATE the JOURNEY

SWALLOW the SUNSHINE

LOCATE that POSITIVE INNER-VOICE

LISTEN to that VOICE

Applying the Senses

Sharp mental health/a healthy mind **smells** like freshly cut grass, lemon zest, or if space had a scent, that's what sharp mental health would **smell** like, open space. Everything about sharp mental health, its **taste, look, and smell,** is open and clean and pure. A blackboard with no chalk marks. A fresh, white sheet of paper. To **touch** sharp mental health is to feel the fleece lining of a protective, waterproof hoodie—it's got you covered no matter what.

Listen? This is what healthy mind sounds like: the rustle of treetops in the woods. A bird's song. A child's giggle. A page turning. Your own first utterance when you were an infant. Sharp mental health and healthy mind **sounds** like a whisper from a trusted friend in an 'I understand, I'm holding space for you.'

All the DEE-5 elements complement each other, they are like a family. Sleep is the eldest, then there's a set of twins - Nutrition and Exercise, and then a younger set, Sharp Mental Health and Tranquil Soul. All different but so closely related.

It is my experience that mental, physical and spiritual health are indelibly linked. If a person experiences a chemical imbalance, their body and their spirit will each display its own kind of imbalance. The interconnectedness of it all is much more complicated than this. Mental health status is directly related to isolation from others, connection to others, and further affected by the stigma associated with mental health disorders. Even the word 'disorder' is an unbalancing and scary word. As humans, loving humans, people supporting people, and as our own best advocates, we have a responsibility to be informed about mental health.

I recognize that writing about mental health issues is a huge responsibility. There are great risks in providing information that could hurt another. For that reason, just like a person without fitness training should be careful in giving fitness direction, someone who does not work in the field of mental health should avoid giving direct advice, yet not shy away from referral, anecdote, or the deep desire to want to help.

To complement the clinical aspects of mental health issues that have been diagnosed as being detrimental to an individual, there are websites, current at the time of writing, which provide solid and professional data. Here are just a few:

- www.mentalhealth.org.uk

- www.apa.org

- ontario.cmha.ca

SHARP MENTAL HEALTH = less stress, balanced scheduling, knowledge

So, What Can We Do to Help Ourselves?

Here is a list of just some of the proven activities and pursuits that can improve mental health situations, stabilize moods, and prevent deterioration:

- Yoga. Participate at least once a week.

- Help your hormones. Consume organic and non-GMO food so that the body can and does support a clear mind.

- Meditate. At least 5-10 minutes (daily). Make it purposed quiet time, focused on breathing.

- Reconnect with nature. Go to the closest area of natural beauty (National Park, Woodland, Protected Reserve, Sanctuary).

- Take breaks. Randomly take 1, 2, or 3 days away from your daily routine to rest the brain, calm the stress, and restore.

- Exercise. Ride a bike, walk, fly a kite. Move and shake your body in different ways compared to a regular workout.

- Research. Locate and engage the support of a psychologist, counsellor, or coach in order to obtain more tools and strategies to face and overcome life's challenges.

- Create an Electronic Sabbath. Choose one day a week to stay away from all electronics.

If you don't feel ready for any of these initiatives yet, commit to staying away from negative social media.

Prioritize your life. Take about 30 minutes to create a current list of priorities. Once that's completed, further prioritize in this exact order:

1) You

2) Family and Friends

3) Business or Work

Supporting the Mental Health of Others

- Plain and simple: Be kind. Be Patient. Be understanding.

- If you find yourself trying to understand how to behave (when you are around someone who has mental health challenges), or if you find yourself unable to empathize, then think about if that person had a visible physical injury. What if that person in front of you evidenced a broken arm, a gunshot wound, a spinal cord injury? Ask yourself, why do I feel differently? Is it because I cannot see the open wounds or scars of mental health?

- Avoid gossiping.

- Stay away from assumptions.

- Explain that you are unfamiliar with words relating to mental health issues and ask the person what bothers him or her.

*****

Q& A Time

"Hey Dee, if I have to reorganize my priorities in order to keep my sanity how can I do it? I am already stressed just thinking about it. My priority right now is to put food on the table for my family." - Joanne

Find ways to make small changes, so small that they don't stress you out. If you find yourself dedicating too much time in your business and not enough time for yourself, being out balance in your priorities is as bad to your health as stress. Let me suggest the following:

1) Book in your calendar 30 minutes a week only for you, make sure that you communicate this to your family, and you are the first person that must respect this without booking anything else as a priority.

2) Book 30 minutes a week of complete undivided attention to your kids or spouse. Make sure that they know about it and also respect your time together.

This might not be flawless at first and after several attempts, be kind and patient with yourself and your family as well.

"Dee, The struggle is real. I am going through a divorce, managing my kids and business all at once. I feel that my body won't be able to handle it for much longer, what can I do?"- Maria

Maria, I understand you because I went through the same situation years ago. Now that I see things more clearly, and having worked with people and worked on myself, I understand now more than ever that taking care of you first is vital. If you don't prioritize yourself, your life situation will only become more insane. Try workouts with a low intensity (see the previous chapter on Complete Exercise). Exercise is proven to help with stress and mental health issues. Eat as healthy as possible, making healthier choices daily. Instead of going to bed with all your issues in your head, place a journal next to your bed, write all the crazy emotions that comes your way and eventually you will be able to sleep with your mind quieter.

"I feel that I am getting angry so easily with the people around me, Dee. I don't feel like I am in control of my emotions or reactions anymore. What can I do?" - Carmen

My dear friend, if you can, take a day off from the city and get some Vitamin N (N for Nature). Nature has the power to balance you, to ground you. Nature has the power to take all the negativity away and renew you 100%.

"Being a single dad is so challenging right now. I feel like I only have enough energy to provide for my kids. I'm trying to keep it all together. When I do have spare time and see my friends again, I'm afraid they won't see me the same way anymore. I don't want to lose myself, but I think it's already happening." – Erick

I get it. As a single mom, I can understand your struggle. It is hard to speak and show your vulnerability but keeping it all to yourself is not doing any good either. Your mental health will suffer. You need your sanity to raise your kids and have a productive and joyful life. If at all possible, I recommend for you to find a babysitter and go play/ connect with your friends as often as you can. Having adult, no-nonsense conversations will help your mind relax and you will return home renewed and refreshed.

Having sharp mental health can be as easy and simple as you make it. When you get to do things that you like, things that bring you joy and make you laugh, (laughter is the best medicine to your heart and mind), you immediately are able to relax the mind and body. This allows your energy to be brought to a higher vibration that recharges you in order to continue with your day to day life.

*****

Reader's Journal

Connect to the *Happy Naked Exclusive Readers'* Resource webpage for downloadable journal pages, links and stay tuned for guided meditations as well. http://deehealthnfitness.com/resources/ - password: 8xxx8

How do I want my mental health to be?

What will I do to make that happen?

Currently, what does my mental health:
Look like:
Sound like:
Smell like:
Taste: like:
Feel like (touch):

What do I want my mental health to:
Look like:
Sound like:
Smell like:
Taste: like:
Feel like (touch):

I will check in next month to see if there are changes in what my mental health looks, sounds, smells, tastes, and feels like. (Put a date in your diary.)

What is the easy fix for me here?

What is the fix I'm shying away from?

(Hint, that's probably the one your mind-body-soul needs you to address.)

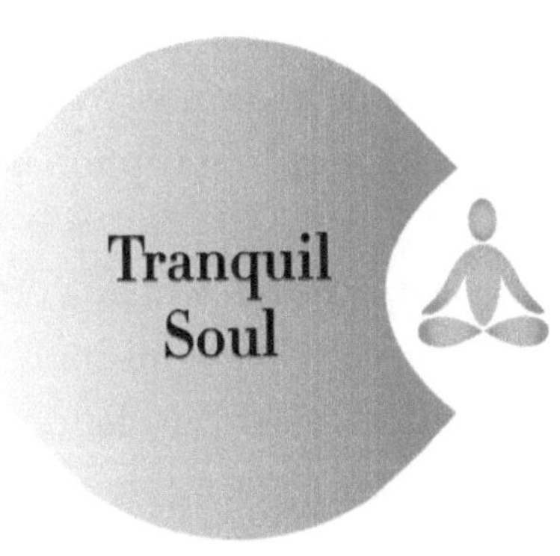

DEE-ism:

Soul: The Other-Worldliness,

And Inner-Worldliness of You.

Applying the Senses

Oh, the **scent** of knowledge. A tranquil soul **smells** like an old forest. It's breathing in the books that are housed in an old library. It's the carved wooden shelves and the rose oil of the person who polished it. It's a sweetness one **tastes** in the air at a welcoming community centre where someone is baking cakes. Tranquil soul **appears** as the powerful surge of a breeching whale. And tranquil soul **sounds** like a Gregorian chant, a gospel choir, a 'welcome home' at one's home-city airport, an eruption of laughter on a busy subway. At its finest, Tranquil Soul is sensed (**touch**) in the feet, through walking on velvety moss. And through the body, Tranquil Soul is like touching a slow dance with love as your dance partner.

TRANQUIL SOUL = spirituality, gratitude, forgiveness, deeper connection

Get To Know Your Soul

What is the soul? Ask a hundred people and you'll get a hundred answers. What do you think? What does soul mean to you?

What are some senses you can associate with the soul?

And if you don't believe there's a soul, then what name do you give that combination of inner-voice, intuition and flame that remains if you remove all the labels associated with you?

Is it an undiscovered organ in the body?

Is it a state of mind?

Is it ever present in every cell?

Is it the higher self?

Is it inner-peace?

Is it faith-based, or even 'religiously' affiliated?

Does it come from somewhere before you're born and go somewhere when your physical body dies?

Now that you've established what you think it might be for you, or what it is for you, here's some of what I find fascinating about conceptions of the soul around the world and through history.

The ancient Egyptians believed each person was made of various elements, physical and spiritual. That's one of the earliest mentions of a soul as a separate part of the body.

There are many faith-based organizations that believe 'the soul' is so connected to God (a creator) that it is 'given,' or 'gifted,' or 'breathed into' a body, and then becomes a part of that person, and continues after their physical death.

In a modern and conventional way of looking at the term 'soul,' and excluding faith-based groups, it would appear that there is an element of 'otherworldly' about the soul. It is a term that basically describes that which we can't describe, or locate, but can feel through our consciousness, through good deed, and through our wanting a better world.

In my view, to be soulful is to be thoughtful. When my soul is healthy, I am connected to that place inside of where I can ask questions. I allow the universe, God, or my inner-voice to guide me, to get me closer to a fulfilling life where my heart, full of love and passion, guides me to serve this planet to be a better place to live.

Latino Zen

I grew up in Venezuela and lived my whole life in such a vibrant culture. Loud, partying all the time, busy and noisy city was my home city of Caracas. Being loud is so ingrained in our DNA that we don't talk, we yell. From a foreigner's perspective, it might look like we are arguing, but it is so not true. We are having a pleasant, lively conversation. My family, I am proud to say, is the loudest in the neighbourhood back home.

When I moved to Canada it was a real culture shock. Not only a different culture and language, but no one yells at anyone here and raising the voice is a sign of disrespect or confrontation. What the heck is that for a Venezuelan? In order for me to adjust in this culture I had to get immersed and learn the way to be myself in this new country. I had to find my inner *Latino Zen*.

First, I had to learn to lower my tone of voice. Second, I had to stop talking with my hands so much as it seemed that Canadian people find that rude. How did I change that? As is often the case, big changes always come in the midst of chaotic times. I was going through massive personal challenges when the path to Latino Zen began. Meditation and yoga were the first things I introduced into my life to become as Zen as a Latina in Canada can be.

Latino Zen is the blending of my super-empowering Fitness Coach role with my energy healing Reiki master training when needed. The Zen in me also shows up in the intimate and vulnerable conversations with my clients.

I have done many practices in the last 10 years of my life as Vipassana, different styles of yoga, Buddhist meditation, Hindu meditation and energy work. Who knew that coming to Canada would take my personal journey down this path?

If you want to see the pure Latino in me, put me in a room full of Venezuelans. In 10 minutes, I am back to talking loudly and with my hands. I am enjoying deafening debates about politics. Believe me, when we finish the party, we are all hugging and kissing like there has been no disagreements at all. This is me: Latino Zen.

Soul-Work

The following are examples of supportive soul-work, which can be called self-love work.

Meditation

Kundalini awakening, regular meditation, compassionate Buddhist meditation, Nidra yoga, listening to guided meditations on YouTube. These are some of the techniques I've engaged to find my inner-voice, peace and guidance and to trust my journey.

Yoga

There are many styles, try them out. Find the one that works for you. I have found that Traditional 26 Hot Yoga is doing exactly what I need in this moment in my life.

Tantra

Most people would link it directly to sex, however, it is about exploring your energy, raising it and learning how to love yourself and connect with people at a deeper level, which can also include sexual or sensual connection. It can be challenging, sometimes uncomfortable, yet worth the results.

Energy Work

Reiki, Shamanic sessions, and hypnosis, will give another level of experience to heal your emotions, and counter those experiences that have created wounds or traumas. When you feel you are 'stuck,' 'blocked,' or have come up against a wall, this kind of energy work is soul-healing.

As a Reiki master, I welcome any reader who wants in-person or distance healing.

Past Life Regression

Removes blocks from specific times in life. It clears patterns that are 'wired' into our being.

Benefits of Soul-Work

When you start putting all the pieces together through any of the soul-work described, initially one can feel overwhelmed.

When we push through the initial overwhelm, you may feel:

- That your life has true purpose

- Healthy and strong

- Your 'cup' is full and you're ready to give back to the world

- Daily gratitude

- Aware of the learning experiences that come from the challenges

- Present, able to live in the now

- Able to trust the future

- Open to all change

- Surrounded by incredibly positive and progressive people

- A measure of self-acceptance

- Accepting of others

*****

Q&A Time

"Meditation is not meant for me. I cannot keep my mind quiet, what can I do?"

You don't have to be a monk to practice meditation. The concept of meditation as it has been taught in the East might not be applicable to you, controlling your thoughts is just one way to meditate.

What I always suggest is to do what you love, do what makes you forget what time it is. Being totally present with something you love doing is a meditative state. Eventually if you wish to get to a deeper connection within yourself, you can join meditation groups and learn some Eastern techniques.

"Dee, I have never experienced energy healing before, Is it actually helpful?"

As a Reiki master, I can tell you from my direct experience that energy work is magic. The energy within you is so powerful, it can heal you, calm you and make you happy in one session. You just need to be open to the experience. It is very common to feel more peaceful at the end of the treatment. Then you will want to come back for more energy work.

"Dear Dee, I don't believe in past lives, so why would I do energy work to connect to past lives for my personal growth or spiritual discovery?"

There are many energy treatments and spiritual guides to explore. Find one that you connect with. You'll know it's the right one when the work allows you to get past the traumas you've experienced and keep growing and evolving as a human being.

*****

Reader's Journal

How do I want my soul to be?

What will I do to make that happen?

Currently, what does my soul:
Look like:
Sound like:
Smell like:
Taste: like:
Feel like (touch):

What do I want my soul to:
Look like:
Sound like:
Smell like:
Taste: like:
Feel like (touch):

I will check in next month to see if there are changes in what my soul looks, sounds, smells, tastes, and feels like. (Put a date in your diary.)

What is the easy fix for me here?

What is the fix I'm shying away from?

Connect to the *Happy Naked Exclusive Readers' Resource* webpage for downloadable journal pages, links and stay tuned for guided meditations as well. You can also book a Reiki session with me through the site. http://deehealthnfitness.com/resources/ - password: 8xxx8

SECTION 3
TYING IT ALL
TOGETHER

Syncronicity

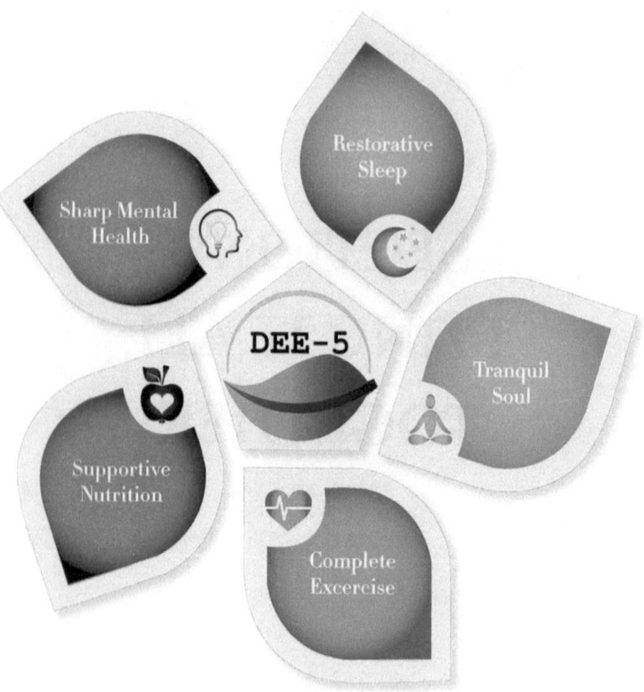

Each section of the DEE-5 System supports each other.

When you bring all five elements into your life, into your pattern of change, you will experience just how thoroughly they support each other. When one area of your health is low, another area will help compensate. For example:

- When feeling stressed, exercise can help the situation.

- When feeling anxious, meditation/yoga/prayer can help.

- When sleep is affected, foods can support the deficit (as can exercise).

- When digestion is an issue, healthy mind and healthy soul-work can provide support to get back on track.

Stopping to evaluate how we are feeling, by using the five senses, further sharpens our awareness of our issues. The latter is absolutely helpful when we use those five senses to describe what we perceive is negative, and then describe its opposite. And, it is extremely healthy when we describe our successes in terms of the five senses.

Building Your Brand of Sensuality

Applying the Senses

Sensuality can look like curves and smooth movement and a glow under the skin. Being happy and confident in your naked body can look like glowing skin at your most natural weight. Sensuality can sound like a calm resonant voice speaking the language of love. Or it can sound like a full-body laugh rising and bringing joy. Sensuality can smell of the sweaty satisfaction of hard work. It can hold the scent of fresh air trapped in your hair smell or of the scent of pure natural clean skin. Sensuality can taste of a ripe fruit savoured slowly and mindfully. And the feeling, sensuality and feeling Happy Naked feels like inner happiness and balance.

What does sensuality mean for you? What are the sensations of feeling sensual for you?

When you are truly *Happy Naked* you will be the most sensual, sexy and confident version of yourself. When you become aware and in touch with your body, your shape will transform, and you will glow with pure health and energy. You will be fully YOU and everyone around you will feel the radiance of your confidence and self-love.

To me, confidence is the most sensual and sexy attribute a person can have. When someone loves the skin they're in, it is hard not to want to be near them. How do you build this kind of confidence? By working with all the DEE-5 elements together, of course! When you put all the Five-to-Thrive into practice, you will enter the positive feedback loop of positive thoughts, feeling healthy, making good choices, feeling happy, and around and around it goes. Health that is felt in all areas of your being will positively impact your hormones, brain functions, mindset, and the beliefs you hold about your own worth and body image.

Happy Naked Fairytales

We all crave stories. Nice once-upon-a-times that have happy endings. It's one of the ways we become inspired to change, to move through our own issues, and to learn. In the spirit of grandmothers sharing stories that inspire us, here are some real people who have inspired me. Each of these *Happy Naked* warriors have used the DEE-5 System elements to find their way to truly becoming *Happy Naked.*

Breanna:

A single mom to three-year-old Riley. Breanna works 8-5 as a file clerk in a busy law office.

She lives in fear of being late. Late for work puts her job in jeopardy. Late for daycare pick-up and she risks her child's placement there. Every workday, after she takes Riley to daycare, Breanna has one hour, in busy traffic, to get from the daycare to work. Then, at the end of a hectic workday, she has another hour in rush hour to get back to the daycare.

She dreads that her child will become sick and has even taken Riley to daycare when he's been a little under the weather. She's used vacation time for when he cannot go.

The pressure Breanna feels from this 'schedule sandwich' is measurable in her tight chest and rushed ways. Unbeknownst to her, this stress pulses through her body and has created some digestive issues.

Her meals are mostly eaten from her child's plate. Her weight has been climbing since Riley was born. Riley sometimes wakes in the night, and at those times, Breanna realizes she, herself, is still up, because after he's in bed, at eight at night, she tunes out of life and into television—late night Netflix binges.

Saturday and Sunday are chaotic catch-ups.

She is not dating, her finances are tight, she never feels like she's getting ahead, and never seems to be available to just stop and think.

There are no activities in her life that she looks forward to. She's in robot mode. She doesn't believe there is any time for living, only for survival. As much as she loves Riley, she is finding herself resentful of parenting. She asks herself where is the joy? She won't even look at herself in the mirror anymore; a ponytail, a pair of black pants and one of five multi-colored tops, and flat shoes—that's her work uniform.

The Catch before the Crash

The law firm announces widespread downsizing is imminent. Breanna believes she'll have some severance when she is laid off, but with the 'break' in employment will also come a job search, let alone a new location, perhaps even further from the daycare.

But, to her surprise, at a meeting with the administrative supervision team, it is expressed how much she is appreciated and needed at the firm.

This confidence buoys her. She's never spoken to her supervisor about her situation—the stress and worry of getting to work, or the guilt of not staying late.

Being open to conversation provides a kind of future lifeline for Breanna. In discussion, one of the admin team talks to Breanna about 'time' and how it will pass quickly, Riley will not always be three.

The senior staff member makes an appointment to meet with Breanna about how the firm can support her. She is an asset to them, and they do not want to lose her.

Changes

That night, with her confidence high, Breanna grabs a paper and pen and orders her priorities.

Me. (without me I cannot be there for my child)

My child.

My job.

The next evening, after work, she left the car outside the daycare and took Riley to a nearby park. She and Riley were hungry, but they had fun and she missed the tail end of the rush hour. Riley slept soundly and Breanna felt a little joy inside.

The next day, she rose early, packed lunches and a bagged supper. And, after daycare, they did the park again. When they arrived home, bath time and bed were a breeze. And no supper dishes to clean.

And so began the path of happiness and health for Breanna. Within a year, she

- Was spending much more time playing outside with Riley than binge-watching TV.

- Wasn't afraid of time anymore, she knew she could handle it.

- Cooked and meal-planned most of their food, and her digestive issues were gone.

- Had inspired a healthy eating and walking movement at her office.

- Exercised everyday whenever possible, even if it was just online yoga or playing with Riley.

- Felt confident in all key areas of her life; able to deal with adversity and be creative with problem-solving.

When we first met Breanna, her life was in chaos—one long uninterrupted chaos. Now she welcomes spontaneity. She feels like she has enough time for work, Riley, and most especially, for herself. She has found her joy.

John:

Used to be a good listener and a passionate doctor. Now, he worries all the time. The clinic he works at has instructed him not to spend so much time listening and to spend more time prescribing medications and seeing as many patients per day as possible.

This is not what he hoped for when he went into medical school. This is not what his grandfather did, nor what his father still does as a rural doctor. John was so proud to get his medical degree and now he is deeply sad and disillusioned.

John has also become his own worst patient. His blood pressure is too high. He has gained so much weight.

He stopped going to the gym. It seemed he had more time when he was in medical school, and that wasn't a lot of time. He is newly married, and he wonders how he and his new wife will be able to spend time together, how he will be a present parent—given the hours he keeps—and he also wonders, if he does have children, how long he'll be around.

All day, Monday to Friday, he writes prescriptions for symptoms, but really wants just to tell people to meditate and exercise, to quit smoking and stop drinking, and to eat good food. But the clinic has expectations and so do patients.

This is not enough. He is not enough. He doesn't want to fight. He's afraid of disappointing others. He knows, above anything, that he needs to get himself healthy so he can be in shape to make decisions that will affect his future, and, quite possibly if not probably, the future of others. He became a doctor to change the face of medicine. He didn't realize the medical system was so flawed, nor did he realize the toll it would take on his body.

Twice in the last week he's almost written his own prescription, (well, asked a trusted colleague to) for something to settle his anxiety.

John Goes Home

John decides that the first thing he must do, is to speak to his new wife, Mary. They'd been together for two years, they are a team. She is creative, they can figure it out together, he figures.

John's good intentions of speaking with Mary left him in shock. After a long conversation one evening, where he poured out his heart, Mary explained, point blank, that part of what attracted her to marrying him was the status of being a doctor's wife. She even said it looked good on her life resume.

John listened; he couldn't respond. She seemed so matter of fact.

John could not focus on any of his patients the whole week. And, by the weekend, he'd spoken to the director of the clinic and put in for a week off.

For solace and space to reflect, John headed to his parents' home in a small northern community. His father, in his late sixties, still delivering medicine to a small town, rural, farming, and indigenous population.

John opens up to his parents. He shares the emotional pain in his heart, and the soullessness he feels in his clinic work. He tells them he's starting to judge other doctors and he knows that's not good.

The next day he sits across the desk from his father in the medical office where John has done many an after-school homework session.

"You first, son," His father says. "It appears I may put my patients first, but I put me first so I can be a good husband, so I can be a good doctor."

"Okay, Pops. Me first."

Pops gave John a *prescription* to help him reconnect to his healthier self. The prescription was to:

- Eat whole foods cooked at home.

- Exercise outside a little every day.

- Attend a sweat lodge and meditate to awaken his spirit.

- Be present to every moment, not worrying about the future.

- Sleep deeply.

- Attend some patients with his dad to awaken his love of medicine.

After hearing the plan, John asked "And then when I go back next week, what do I do?"

"Decide that on Sunday, son. Live in the now."

"Or else?" John asked.

"There is no "or else." I'm saving your life. And, son, I don't want you to give in to any pressure from anyone. You need to do what you need to do. What your heart tells you to do."

And so, full of faith in his father's plan, John dove in. He fulfilled the prescription and then some.

A Knight in Shining Sneakers

Fast forward one year. John, fifty pounds lighter in body and soul, has a small office in the main floor of what used to be a crack house. There are rooms upstairs for transitional housing. A social worker, a psychologist, a public health nurse, and an administrator work together with John. 'Not Your Ordinary Doctor" is funded by three faith-based groups, who keep their faith names out of the title. John goes into his old clinic twice a week to meet with old staff, to convince them to get on board with changing the way medicine is delivered.

The emergency room at the hospital has seen a decrease in use and overuse by some of the marginalized population of the inner city. 'Not Your Ordinary Doctor' has impacted care through community outreach.

John's divorce will be finalized next month. His ex-wife is dating a litigation lawyer. Her sister told John she's regretful of their breakup because John is now being recognized by the Mayor and City council.

John wears running shoes all the time - from Fields. He exercises regularly and has climbed to the summit of Chinook Mountain three times since his original visit to his parents. He's currently putting together a group retreat for doctors who are stressed out. They'll visit the mountain and attend a sweat lodge.

John is content: he exercises, eats healthy food, sleeps like a baby, has work that feeds soul, and honors himself to maintain his mental health. He is most definitely Happy Naked.

Helen

Is a successful realtor with three teen kids. Her husband, Harry, is a civil engineer with a large development firm. The kids are heavily scheduled with after-school activities. Helen feels like she has to always be *on*. Her calendar is packed, she misses meals and has no time for friends. She spends her dollars on random *stuff* because she doesn't know how else to have a presence in her life. She feels like a very well decked-out hamster on a wheel.

She is more focused on being there for her clients than for her family. It seems to have just slowly become that way. Helen and her husband make great money, more than most couples, but at the end of the month she probably has less than most. There are simply so many fees associated with all their activities and maintenance for all their material possessions.

They eat out most of the time. Despite her household income, Helen feels poor in spirit. She wants the best but can't understand what that 'best' is. Helen longs for quality time because she's heard that phrase and aches for *something* but doesn't know what 'quality time' really is. Her marriage feels disconnected, yet to others it looks great. They are Mr. and Mrs. Dance parents. Mr. and Mrs. Hockey parents. They are professionals and they have letters after their names.

What about exercise? She's running around all day, but it's all done by sitting in her car.

Meditation? That's for trippy people who have checked out of life, live in caves and communes.

Sleep? The sofa bed is the best money can buy and it's so close to the computer, the phone, the tablet and the back-up cell phone.

Food? Restaurants. Only the finest and all those lovely sandwiches with organic ingredients made by a local café, with a Frappuccino, of course. A girl's gotta hydrate.

Helen is running close to empty. Financially. Energetically. Spiritually. She's a good person who is out of control.

Crisis

And then, it happens. No, not a crash in the real estate market. Worse. Helen's husband has a heart attack.

She thought she was overscheduled before? Harry will stay in for some more tests and observation. There are three hockey games this weekend, a dance recital, an open house and an offer on one of her properties. She pays a fortune for parking at the hospital. She sits by Harry's bed. Then she's cut off, no charge in her cell phone. She's forced to sit idle while Harry sleeps.

Out of boredom, she wanders the halls and finds the chapel. Without thinking, she opens the plain wooden door. There are chairs in rows, soft light flows though the mostly open space. There are no people in here. It is so silent.

She sits.

She breathes.

She never wants to leave this room.

She drifts off to sleep, sitting up. Helen startles awake when someone opens the door. She watches a man take a seat and close his eyes. She gets up and leaves and promises the door she'll be back.

Next day, she returns to the chapel. The man is gone. There are two women, she makes three. She sits in silence. No one speaks, only breathing can be heard.

Helen's Soul-Work Begins

With a heavy reliance on the help of others to take her children to dance and hockey, Helen focuses on taking back control of the family finances. When she visits Harry in the hospital, she goes to the chapel. She finds peace there every time.

She sets up a meeting with their accountant and is beyond shocked to find out how much debt they have.

She attends the hospital exercise classes with Harry, as well as the cooking instructions. Finally, she moves him home, into their bedroom.

She talks to the kids about reducing their activities. They actually seem relieved.

She finds a junior in the office to help her and arranges a commission split. The freedom is incredible.

Every little creative thing she can do, she does. It helps others and it helps her: Win-win.

And she continues to go to the chapel. Such joy enters her life when it is quiet.

Lives Happily Ever After

A year later, Helen is in the top twenty in her office. Harry is back at work. Only one boy is in hockey. The other has been volunteering at the SPCA and works at a coffee shop part time. He loves it. Her daughter is dancing and has received a scholarship to a prominent university known for fine arts.

Helen and Harry have discussed in detail how their lives used to be. They are even grateful for the heart attack. They wonder if it would have been wiser to declare bankruptcy—their debt repayment schedule has been more challenging than difficult. After all, they make great money.

There are no more Amazon deliveries that arrive at their door. Helen has let her hair grey naturally. Harry loves it. They walk. They even speak at the wellness classes that they once participated in—guest speakers at the orientation for others on wellness journeys (forced wellness journeys).

Tracking Your Happy Naked Life

You can only know how far you've come if you track where you start and where you have been. And if you've worked your way through the exercises in these chapters, I have no doubt you have come a long way indeed!

Throughout this book, each section of the DEE-5 System has called you to journal about your progress and your experiences. The very act of reflecting and recording strengthens and solidifies your transformation. You may have times when it might seem like too much effort to track your efforts and progress.

Tracking is essential to sustainable long-term change, because there's no other way to learn exactly what's working for you and what is not. Your body may be challenged by exercise for a time and then plateau. Without tracking your efforts and progress, you may not notice when a new habit is no longer enough challenge for you.

The very most valuable result of journaling and tracking is that it builds a strong habit of putting yourself first and being attentive to your overall wellbeing. This is about taking control of your health and fitness and loving the skin you're in—for good!

Recommendation

Please write in your journal, keep it and review once in a while to reflect on your progress. This is not about perfection in journaling: it's about the act itself, not perfecting your writing skills.

In each of your journal entries, especially when you are not sure what to write, go to the senses: what does today taste like, sound like, feel like, look like, and smell like?

Create the habit of journaling which will allow you to develop self-discipline when it comes to life balance.

I would be so grateful if you want to share your story of shift, glow and confidence with me. Reach out to me, I truly want to know about your journey and how this book benefits your overall health and fitness.

THE END OF THIS BOOK

IS THE

THE CONNECTION OF US

IS THE

THE BEGINNING OF YOU

"We but mirror the world.
All the tendencies present in the outer world
are to be found in the world of our body.
If we could change ourselves,
the tendencies in the world would also change.
As a man changes his own nature,
so does the attitude of the world change towards him.
This is the divine mystery supreme.
A wonderful thing it is and the source of
our happiness.
We need not wait to see what others do."

Mahatma Gandhi

Acknowledgements

With deep gratitude:

Mom. You provided a home which has allowed me financial freedom to follow my dreams and passions to inspire, motivate, and transform people through conscious living. I am so grateful.

Grandma. You're the warrior who has shown me strength, pure love, family closeness, and support...all without judgement. Gracias Abuelita.

My awesome kids consistently support me: Deborah, Valery, and Hector you are my biggest fans. Kids – know this: I am yours.

Oscar, my former husband: You showed me the beauty and importance of communication.

Luc, you taught me how to live my life without judgement, to be open to love and life, and to ask questions in order understand the situations of others.

At the risk of missing some individuals, this book has been influenced by many I consider my teachers, mentors, and friends: Bruce Cruickshank and Colin

Sprake; Andrea Thatcher and Debra Kasowski, you are both key players to me following my dream; Ehlana Mohamed a sweet yoga instructor, very passionate and awesome friend; James Kirouac with his incredible passion to change the world; Joanne Prystay such a loyal friend and supporter; Jorge Szeoke and Mariela Parra, they're true believers; Marcel Hertzfeldt, an extraordinary friend; Milvia Rodriguez, such an inspiration; Natalie Kae Samanco, a great friend with passion for yoga and mental health; Octavio Toro, your passion for plant-based eating habits and health is enormous; Rovena Skye changed my life and taught me so many new things in my personal life that I can apply everywhere—grateful am I to have found a real and passionate teacher in the tantric world; Wael Badawy, I cannot thank you enough for all the learning and support.

This book could not have been prepared without the incredible help of Marie Beswick-Arthur. Thank you for being the best editor ever.

The list could go on and on...

This project could not happen without having a healthy body and a fulfilling life.

In the end, A BIG THANKS TO LIFE. Life is more than looking good naked. We need to touch, hear, taste, listen, and see the glory of our human-ness and what it is like to be *Happy Naked*.

About the Author

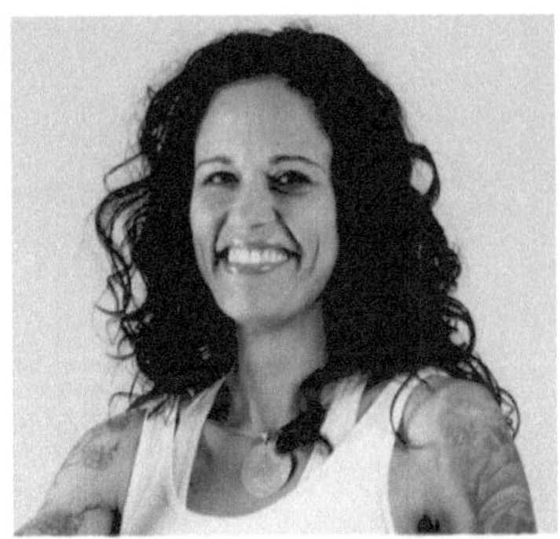

If passion and spunk had a love child – that would be Dee Mago.

Founder of Dee Health n' Fitness, Dee Mago's zesty blend of Latin Zen + Naked Truth has been keeping her one-on-one clients and class participants energized and inspired for over 5 years.

A dynamic Certified Personal Trainer, Reiki master, Healthy Eating Coach, and iFLow teacher, Dee has taught hundreds of people how to move from ashamed of their health to feeling truly happy naked.

Dee Mago lives in Calgary with her three children. 'Happy Naked' is her first (but not last) book.